Atlas of Surgical Approaches to Soft Tissue and Oncologic Diseases in the Dog and Cat

Atlas of Surgical Approaches to Soft Tissue and Oncologic Diseases in the Dog and Cat

Marije Risselada, DVM, PhD, DECVS, DACVS-SA
Department of Veterinary Clinical Sciences
Purdue University College of Veterinary Medicine
West Lafayette
IN, USA

Illustrations by Alice MacGregor Harvey

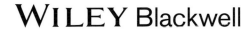

Registered Office
John Wiley & Sons, Inc., 111 River Street, Hoboken, NJ 07030, USA

Editorial Office
111 River Street, Hoboken, NJ 07030, USA

For details of our global editorial offices, customer services, and more information about Wiley products visit us at www.wiley.com.

Wiley also publishes its books in a variety of electronic formats and by print-on-demand. Some content that appears in standard print versions of this book may not be available in other formats.

Library of Congress Cataloging-in-Publication Data

Names: Risselada, Marije, 1973- author.
Title: Atlas of surgical approaches to soft tissue and oncologic diseases in the dog and cat / Marije Risselada ; illustrations by Alice MacGregor Harvey.
Description: Hoboken, NJ : Wiley-Blackwell, 2020.
Identifiers: LCCN 2020017962 (print) | LCCN 2020017963 (ebook) | ISBN 9781119370130 (cloth) | ISBN 9781119370178 (adobe pdf) | ISBN 9781119370192 (epub)
Subjects: MESH: Dog Diseases–surgery | Cat Diseases–surgery | Surgical Procedures, Operative–veterinary | Neoplasms–veterinary | Neoplasms–surgery | Atlas
Classification: LCC SF992.C35 (print) | LCC SF992.C35 (ebook) | NLM SF 992.C35 | DDC 636.089/6994–dc23
LC record available at https://lccn.loc.gov/2020017962
LC ebook record available at https://lccn.loc.gov/2020017963

Cover Design: Wiley
Cover Images: Illustration credit – Alice MacGregor Harvey

Set in 9.5/12.5pt STIXTwoText by SPi Global, Pondicherry, India
Printed and bound in Singapore by Markono Print Media Pte Ltd

10   9   8   7   6   5   4   3   2   1

Contents

Section 3   Forelimb   *101*

Section 4   Hindlimb   *123*

Section 5   Thorax   *155*

Section 6   Abdomen   *189*

Section 7   Perineal Area and Pelvic Canal   *227*

Section 8   Digits and Tail   *253*

Preface

My goal in creating this book was to generate a go-to atlas that any starting surgeon or surgeon-in-training could use as a guide in preparing for soft tissue and oncologic cases or as a resource in the operating room to complement existing atlases. Several novel approaches and new procedures have been published in the veterinary scientific literature in the last several years; although most have been described in textbooks, no specific illustrated atlas incorporating these updated approaches and procedures has existed until now.

Included are chapters on oromaxillofacial approaches as well as the cervical area and ear, forelimb, hindlimb, thorax, and abdomen. The book finishes with approaches to the perineal area, pelvic canal, and digits and tail. Its thoroughness makes this atlas an excellent guide for planning and executing approaches to soft tissue and oncologic diseases.

It is my hope that this book will serve future veterinarians, surgeons, and surgeons-in-training to facilitate learning new procedures or quickly brushing up prior to surgery.

Marije Risselada
West-Lafayette, IN, USA

Section 1
Oromaxillofacial

Approach to the Rostral Mandible[1]

INDICATIONS

- Partial mandibulectomy
- Rostral mandibulectomy
- Lip avulsion repair

PATIENT POSITIONING AND DESCRIPTION OF THE PROCEDURE

I) The lips are clipped and the skin is aseptically prepped and the oral cavity prepared for surgery. The patient is placed in ventral/sternal recumbency with the maxilla suspended by surgical tape, allowing the mandible to hang down in a natural position with the entire mandible draped in.

II) The margins around the neoplastic lesion are measured and marked with a sterile marker. The labial and oral mucosa are incised along the preplanned line using a blade. Stay sutures, skin hooks, or retractors can be used to elevate the lip away from the surgical field. A periosteal elevator is used to free the bone from muscular and fibrous attachments.

   A stab incision is made caudal to the symphysis. The defect is enlarged by blunt elevation and sharp dissection with a periosteal elevator and/or scissors to allow the caudal osteotomies to be made without soft tissue trauma.

   Bone wax or a hemoclip can be used to stop the bleeding from the mandibular alveolar artery after completing the caudal cut.

Atlas of Surgical Approaches to Soft Tissue and Oncologic Diseases in the Dog and Cat, First Edition. Marije Risselada.
© 2020 John Wiley & Sons, Inc. Published 2020 by John Wiley & Sons, Inc.

Approach to the Rostral Mandible

I)

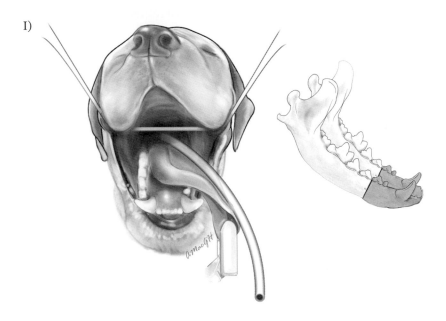

II)

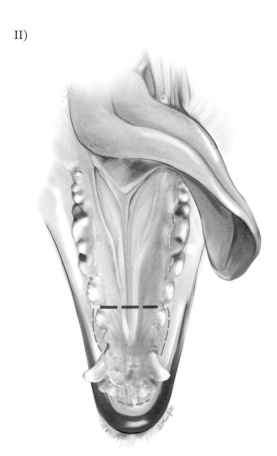

PATIENT POSITIONING AND DESCRIPTION OF THE PROCEDURE *continued*

III) The excess rostral lip is trimmed in a triangle with the base oriented rostrally. The edges of the lip are moved towards the dorsal midline (A to A and B to B) to start the closure.

CLOSURE

The closure is started by assessing if excess lip needs to be trimmed; it is continued by approximating the deeper layers if possible and performing a simple interrupted or simple continuous closure of the mucosa (labial mucosa to the gingiva on each side of midline). The lip (the defect left from the triangle removed at the rostral aspect) is closed in three layers: mucosa, muscle/connective tissue, skin.

   If the cut was through the symphysis, bone tunnels can be drilled to anchor the soft tissues of the lip to the bone with suture.

ALTERNATE POSITIONING AND APPROACHES

- An alternative to a hanging drape is to place the dog in dorsal recumbency with the head and neck elevated on a sandbag/towel with the entire mandible draped in.

Approach to the Rostral Mandible *continued*

III)

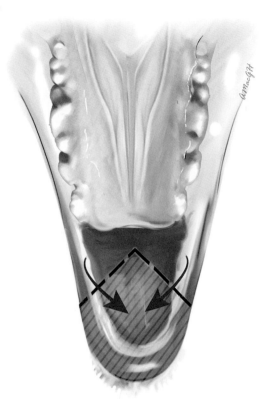

Ventral Approach to the Ramus of the Mandible[2]

INDICATIONS

- Ventral approach to the mandibular bone

PATIENT POSITIONING AND DESCRIPTION OF THE PROCEDURE

I) The patient is placed in dorsal recumbency with the neck extended. The mandibular area, extending as needed into the cervical area, is clipped and prepped. A sandbag or towel can be placed under the neck of the patient to stabilize the head. The legs are pulled backwards. The maxilla can be taped down to the table, increasing the stability of positioning. The mouth can be positioned open during preparation, allowing the entire mandible to be draped into the surgical field if needed.

II) The skin incision is centered over the mandibular ramus, running parallel to the horizontal ramus of the mandible. The subcutaneous tissues are bluntly dissected to expose the digastricus muscle. The digastricus muscle is either transected at a point away from the bone (for margins) or dissected off the bone with a periosteal elevator if no margins are required.

CLOSURE

The incision is closed by approximating the deeper tissues, subcutaneous layer, and skin in an appositional fashion.

ALTERNATE POSITIONING AND APPROACHES

- A midline incision centered between the mandibular rami allows access to the tongue base without entering the oral cavity.

Atlas of Surgical Approaches to Soft Tissue and Oncologic Diseases in the Dog and Cat, First Edition. Marije Risselada.
© 2020 John Wiley & Sons, Inc. Published 2020 by John Wiley & Sons, Inc.

Ventral Approach to the Ramus of the Mandible

I)

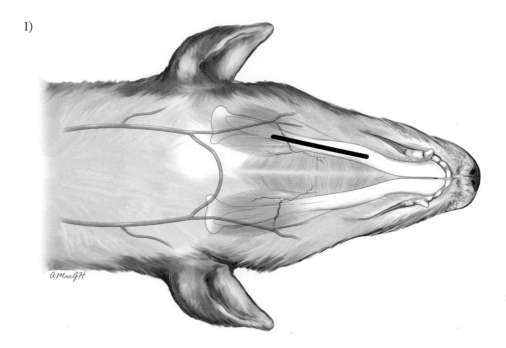

II)

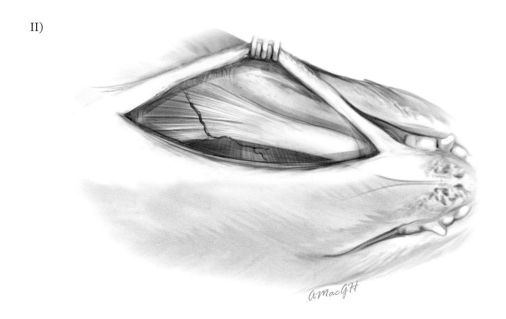

Intraoral Approach to the Ramus of the Mandible[2,3]

INDICATIONS

- Segmental mandibulectomy

PATIENT POSITIONING AND DESCRIPTION OF THE PROCEDURE

I) The patient is placed in lateral recumbency with the upper and lower lips clipped, prepped, and draped in. The lateral cervical area can be draped in as well to allow for access to the mandibular lymph node or for an advancement flap for closure of the defect if needed. A sterile mouth gag can be placed on the down side to maintain access to the oral cavity without the need for manual retraction of the mandible.

   The margins around the neoplastic lesion are measured and marked with a sterile marker. The labial and oral mucosa are incised along the preplanned line using a blade. Stay sutures, a skin hook, or retractors can be used to elevate the lip away from the surgical field.

II) On the oral surface, the mylohyoideus muscle caudally and the geniohyoideus muscle rostrally are elevated from the bone using a periosteal elevator, taking care not to damage the salivary gland and duct.

Intraoral Approach to the Ramus of the Mandible

I)

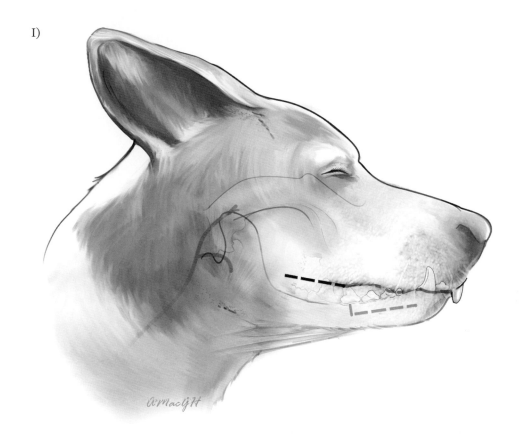

II)

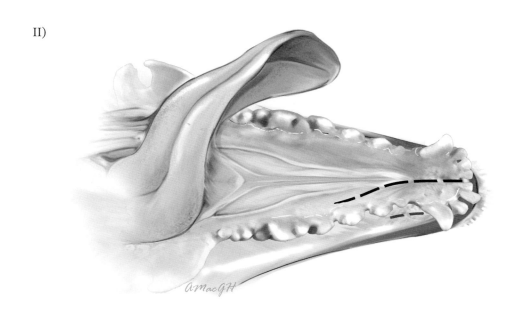

PATIENT POSITIONING AND DESCRIPTION OF THE PROCEDURE *continued*

III)   Labially, the digastricus muscle is elevated away from the bone, allowing access to the preplanned osteotomy site. The osteotomies can be performed with a high speed drill, an osteotome and mallet, or an oscillating saw.

IV)   Depending on the size and location of the lesion, the rostral cut can be at the symphysis, caudal to the ipsilateral canine or across the midline. Bone wax or a hemoclip can be used to stop the bleeding from the mandibular alveolar artery after completing the caudal cut.

CLOSURE

This is performed by approximating the deeper layers first and performing a simple interrupted or simple continuous closure of the mucosa.

ALTERNATE POSITIONING AND APPROACHES

- For a full mandibulectomy the incision is extended caudally, with a full thickness commissurotomy to allow access to the vertical ramus of the mandible (see Lateral Approach to the Mandible).

Intraoral Approach to the Ramus of the Mandible *continued*

III)

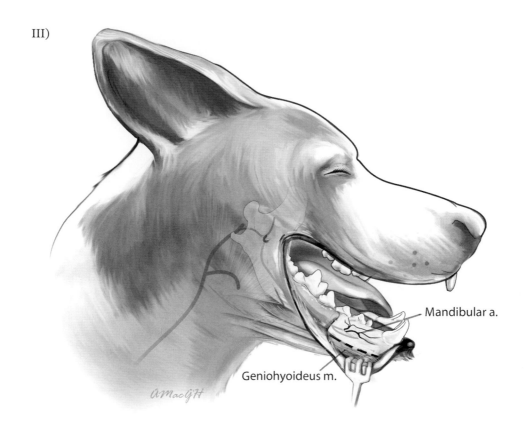

Mandibular a.

Geniohyoideus m.

IV)

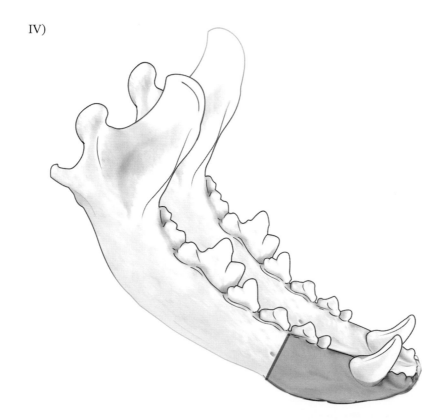

Lateral Approach to the Mandible[1,3]

INDICATIONS

- Mandibular rim excision
- Segmental mandibulectomy
- Mandibulectomy

PATIENT POSITIONING AND DESCRIPTION OF THE PROCEDURE

I) The patient is placed in lateral recumbency with the upper and lower lips clipped, prepped, and draped in. The lateral cervical area can be draped in as well to allow commissurotomy and for access to the mandibular lymph node or for an advancement flap for closure of the defect if needed. A sterile mouth gag can be placed on the down side to maintain access to the oral cavity without the need for manual retraction.

   The margins around the neoplastic lesion are measured and marked with a sterile marker.

II) A full thickness incision is made at the commissure to allow exposure of the vertical ramus of the mandible. The labial and oral mucosa are incised along the preplanned line using a blade. Stay sutures or retractors can be used to elevate the lip away from the surgical field.

   On the oral surface, the mylohyoideus muscle caudally and the geniohyoideus muscle rostrally are elevated from the bone using a periosteal elevator, taking care not to damage the salivary gland and duct. Labially, the digastricus muscle is elevated away from the bone. The masseter muscle overlies the vertical ramus of the mandible and is cut at its ventral attachment and elevated dorsally to expose the dorsal extent of the mandible and the approach to the temporomandibular joint.

Atlas of Surgical Approaches to Soft Tissue and Oncologic Diseases in the Dog and Cat, First Edition. Marije Risselada.
© 2020 John Wiley & Sons, Inc. Published 2020 by John Wiley & Sons, Inc.

Lateral Approach to the Mandible

I)

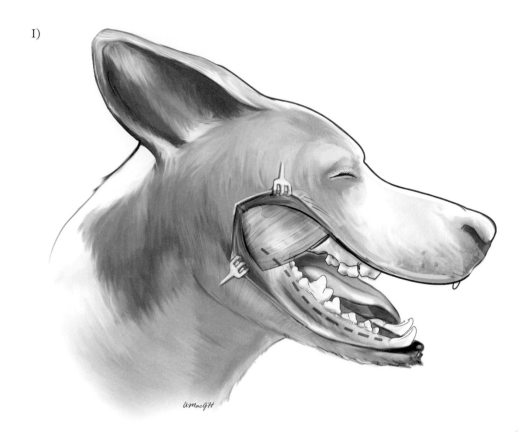

II)

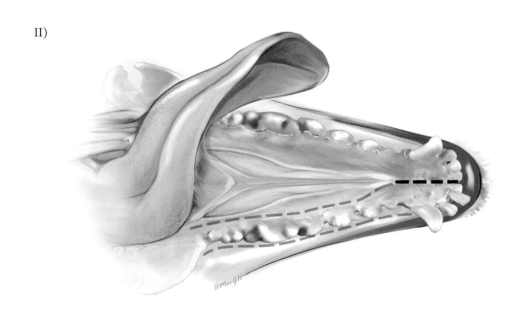

PATIENT POSITIONING AND DESCRIPTION OF THE PROCEDURE *continued*

III) The osteotomies can be performed with a high speed drill, an osteotome and mallet, or an oscillating saw. For a full mandibulectomy, the rostral cut is typically at the symphysis (but can be altered depending on the location of the lesion) and is performed first to allow lateral retraction of the mandible. The pterygoid muscle, located medial to the vertical ramus, is severed last to allow removal of the left or right mandible.

CLOSURE

This is performed by approximating the deeper layers first in an interrupted or continuous suture pattern, followed by performing a simple interrupted or simple continuous closure of the mucosa.

The commissure is closed in three layers: mucosa, muscle, skin. The commissure can be advanced cranially to decrease deviation of the tongue and/or drooling. The closure can be reinforced by placing a button or stent on the dorsal and ventral side at the commissure to avoid the incision lines pulling apart by opening the mouth.

Lateral Approach to the Mandible *continued*

III)

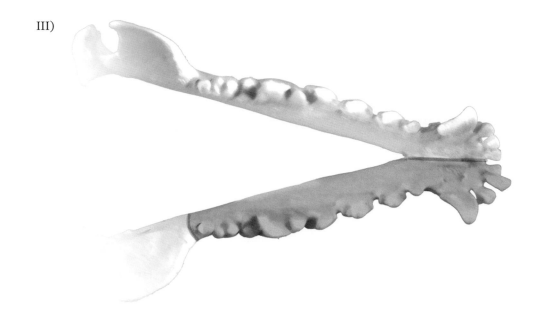

Nasal Planectomy and Premaxillectomy in the Dog[4-7]

INDICATIONS

- Nasal planum tumors with bony involvement
- Rostral maxillary tumors

PATIENT POSITIONING AND DESCRIPTION OF THE PROCEDURE

I, II) The entire maxilla is clipped and prepped and the patient is placed in ventral recumbency with the head and neck elevated on a sandbag/towel with the maxilla draped in. A drape can be placed in the oral cavity or the mandible can be draped in. Margins are planned around the tumor and can be outlined with a sterile marker.

Atlas of Surgical Approaches to Soft Tissue and Oncologic Diseases in the Dog and Cat, First Edition. Marije Risselada.
© 2020 John Wiley & Sons, Inc. Published 2020 by John Wiley & Sons, Inc.

Nasal Planectomy and Premaxillectomy in the Dog

I)

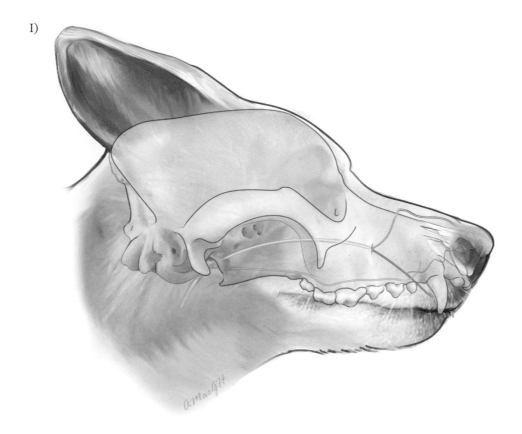

II)

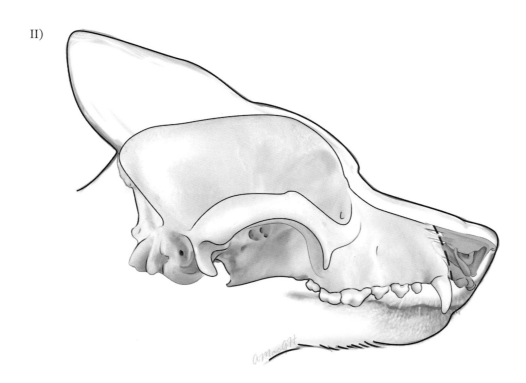

PATIENT POSITIONING AND DESCRIPTION OF THE PROCEDURE *continued*

III) An external skin incision is made along the planned excision line and is extended full thickness through the upper lip bilaterally to connect to the intraoral part of the resection.

Internally, an incision is made through the mucosa and the soft tissues are elevated off the bone with a periosteal elevator, exposing the bone along the preplanned osteotomy line. The osteotomy can be performed with an osteotome and mallet, oscillating saw, high speed air drill, or a combination.

Turbinates are broken down by blunt and sharp dissection and the rostral maxilla removed. Bleeding can be stopped by direct pressure, gauze soaked in cold saline, or hemostatic agents. If bleeding persists from the palatine artery, ligation might be necessary.

CLOSURE

IV) The labial submucosa + mucosa are attached to the gingival and palatine bone, periosteum, and mucosa in a single layer appositional suture pattern. Bone tunnels can be used to secure the submucosal layer to the bone. The left and right lip are brought together (arrows) to allow reconstruction of the lip.

V) The free edges of the rostral edges of the lip are closed in a three layer pattern (mucosa, submucosa, skin) to close the oral cavity. The knots of the mucosal sutures can be buried within the closure if absorbable suture is used, allowing for easier visualization of the suture line. Lastly the skin is reattached to the nasal passages (to periosteum, bone, or cartilage) to create a new nasal orifice. This can be done in a simple interrupted or a simple continuous suture pattern.

ALTERNATE POSITIONING AND APPROACHES

- This approach can involve a nasal planectomy only or can involve a combination of a nasal planectomy with a rostral maxillectomy.
- If only a nasal planectomy is performed, reconstruction is similar, and follows V.
- An alternate approach, if the nasal planum or skin are not included in the resection, is to position the patient in dorsal recumbency with the lips falling away from the maxilla.

Nasal Planectomy and Premaxillectomy in the Dog *continued*

III)

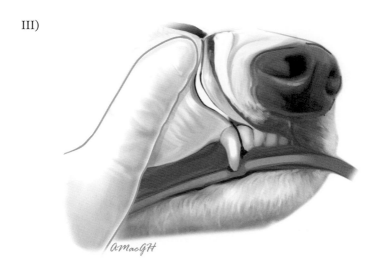

IV)

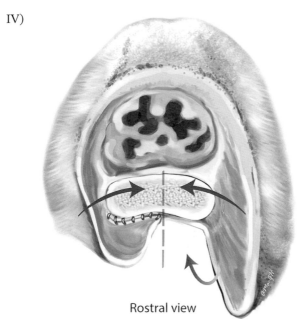

Rostral view

V)

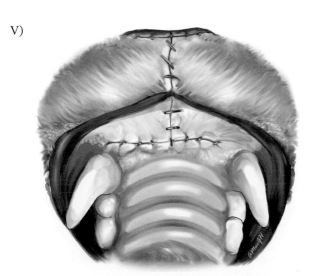

Nasal Planectomy in the Cat[4-6]

INDICATIONS

- Nasal planum tumors

PATIENT POSITIONING AND DESCRIPTION OF THE PROCEDURE

I) The patient is placed in ventral recumbency with the head and neck elevated on a sandbag/towel with the maxilla draped in. A drape can be placed in the oral cavity or the mandible can be draped in. Margins are planned around the tumor and can be outlined with a sterile marker.

II) An external skin incision is made along the planned excision line and is extended full thickness. The soft tissues are elevated off the bone with a periosteal elevator, exposing the bone. Bleeding can be stopped by direct pressure, gauze soaked in cold saline, or hemostatic agents.

CLOSURE

This is achieved by suturing the skin to the nasal passages (to periosteum, bone, or cartilage) to create a new nasal orifice. This can be done in a simple interrupted or a simple continuous suture pattern.

Atlas of Surgical Approaches to Soft Tissue and Oncologic Diseases in the Dog and Cat, First Edition. Marije Risselada.
© 2020 John Wiley & Sons, Inc. Published 2020 by John Wiley & Sons, Inc.

Nasal Planectomy in the Cat

I)

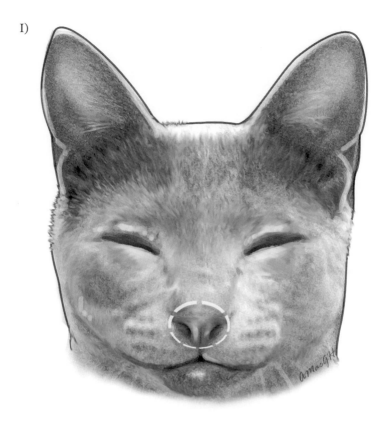

II)

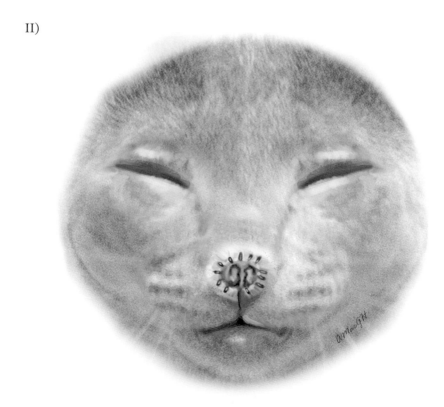

Approach to the Rostral Maxilla[1,3,8]

INDICATIONS

- Rostral maxillary neoplastic or traumatic lesion

PATIENT POSITIONING AND DESCRIPTION OF THE PROCEDURE

I, II) The patient is placed in dorsal recumbency with the head and neck elevated on a sandbag/towel with the mandible and maxilla draped in.

   The margins around the neoplastic lesion are measured and marked with a sterile marker. The labial mucosa and hard palate mucosa and periosteum are incised along the preplanned line using a blade. Stay sutures or retractors can be used to elevate the lip away from the surgical field.

Atlas of Surgical Approaches to Soft Tissue and Oncologic Diseases in the Dog and Cat, First Edition. Marije Risselada.
© 2020 John Wiley & Sons, Inc. Published 2020 by John Wiley & Sons, Inc.

Approach to the Rostral Maxilla

I)

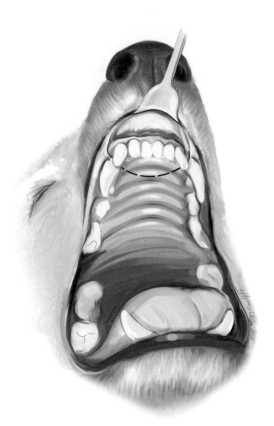

II)

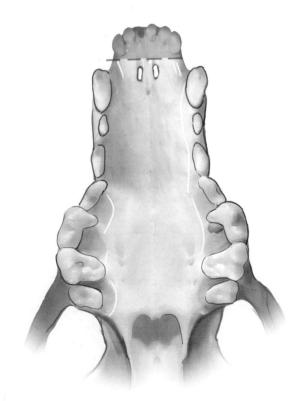

PATIENT POSITIONING AND DESCRIPTION OF THE PROCEDURE *continued*

III) The palatine periosteum and mucosa are elevated caudally using a periosteal elevator until the bone is exposed along the entirety of the planned excision. The osteotomy can be performed with an osteotome and mallet, oscillating saw, high speed drill, or a combination. Turbinates are broken down by blunt and sharp dissection and the rostral maxilla removed. Bleeding can be stopped by direct pressure, gauze soaked in cold saline, or hemostatic agents. If bleeding persists from the palatine artery, ligation might be necessary. Bone tunnels are drilled in the palatine bone to anchor the lip to the bone. The submucosa is attached to the bone in simple interrupted sutures.

CLOSURE

IV) The mucosa is sutured to the periosteal layer in a simple interrupted or a simple continuous suture pattern.

ALTERNATE POSITIONING AND APPROACHES

- An alternative is to place the dog in ventral/sternal recumbency with the maxilla suspended by surgical tape, or with the head elevated on a sandbag and the mouth propped open.
- If the lesion extends to the nasal planum, then a combination of a rostral maxillectomy with a nasal planectomy might be necessary (see Nasal Planectomy and Premaxillectomy in the Dog).

Approach to the Rostral Maxilla *continued*

III)

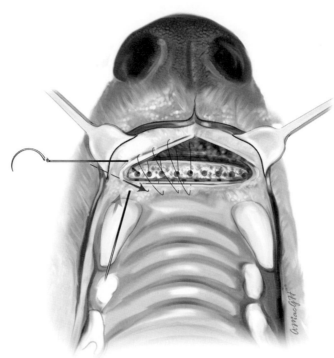

IV)

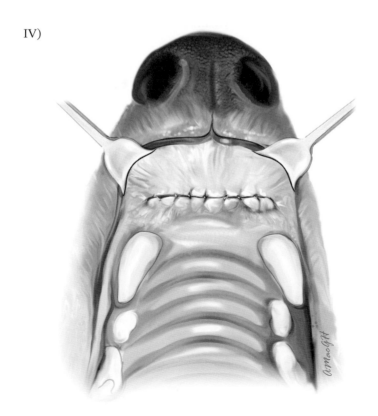

Intraoral Approach to the Maxilla[3]

INDICATIONS

- Segmental maxillectomy
- Partial maxillectomy
- Caudal maxillectomy

PATIENT POSITIONING AND DESCRIPTION OF THE PROCEDURE

I) The patient is placed in lateral recumbency with the lateral cervical area and the upper lip clipped, prepped, and draped in. The lower aspect of the lateral cervical area can be draped in as well to allow for access to the mandibular lymph node or for an advancement flap for closure of the defect if needed. A sterile mouth guard can be placed to maintain access to the oral cavity without the need for manual retraction.

II) The margins around the neoplastic lesion are measured and marked with a sterile marker. Stay sutures or retractors can be used to elevate the lip away from the surgical field. The labial and oral mucosa over the hard palate are incised along the preplanned line using a blade. A periosteal elevator is used to dissect the gingival and labial mucosa away laterally and the palatine periosteum and mucosa medially until the bone is exposed along the entirety of the planned osteotomy line.

Atlas of Surgical Approaches to Soft Tissue and Oncologic Diseases in the Dog and Cat, First Edition. Marije Risselada.
© 2020 John Wiley & Sons, Inc. Published 2020 by John Wiley & Sons, Inc.

Intraoral Approach to the Maxilla

I)

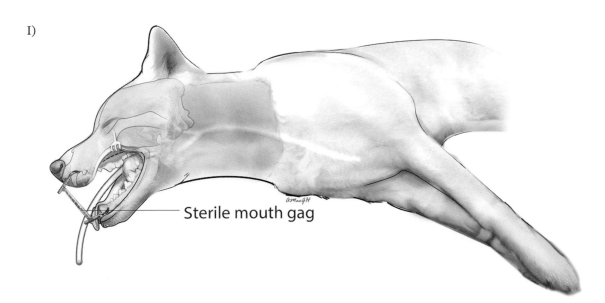

Sterile mouth gag

II)

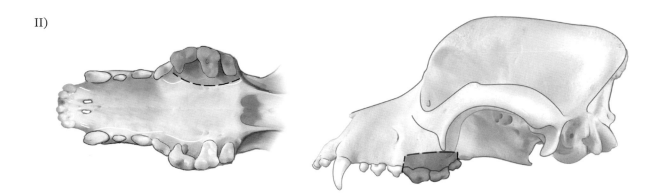

PATIENT POSITIONING AND DESCRIPTION OF THE PROCEDURE *continued*

III) The osteotomy can be performed with an osteotome and mallet, oscillating saw, high speed drill, or a combination. Turbinates are broken down by blunt and sharp dissection and the rostral maxilla removed. Bleeding from the hard palate and turbinates can be stopped by direct pressure, gauze soaked in cold saline, or hemostatic agents. If bleeding persists from the palatine artery, ligation or hemoclip application might be necessary.

CLOSURE

A two layer closure is performed if possible: submucosa to the palatine periosteum in the deep layer and mucosa to mucosa in a separate layer. Bone tunnels can be drilled to anchor the submucosa to the palatine bone and periosteum if any tension is appreciated during closure. The mucosal closure can be a simple interrupted or a simple continuous closure pattern.

ALTERNATE POSITIONING AND APPROACHES

- Depending on the location of the lesion, the incisions will be centered more rostrally to include incisors, the canine, and premolars.
- A very caudal lesion might be easier to approach and visualize using a combined dorsolateral and intraoral approach (see Combined Dorsolateral and Intraoral Approach to the Caudal Maxilla).

Intraoral Approach to the Maxilla *continued*

III)

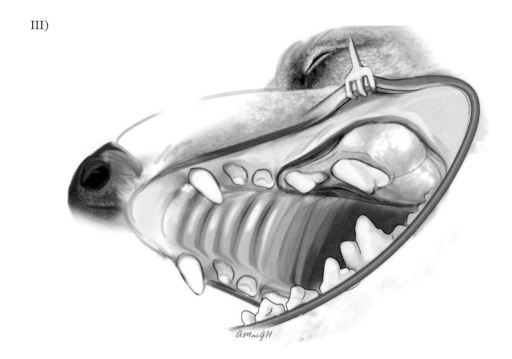

Combined Dorsolateral and Intraoral Approach to the Caudal Maxilla[9]

INDICATIONS

- Caudal maxillary tumors
- Maxillectomy with or without orbitectomy

PATIENT POSITIONING AND DESCRIPTION OF THE PROCEDURE

I) The patient is placed in lateral recumbency with the lateral cervical area and the upper lip clipped, prepped, and draped in. The head is stabilized and elevated on a sandbag/towel and the legs are pulled back. A sterile mouth gag can be placed on the down side to maintain access to the oral cavity without the need for manual retraction.

   The lower aspect of the lateral cervical area can be draped in as well to allow for access to the mandibular lymph node or for an advancement flap for closure of the defect if needed.

II) A skin incision is made ventral to the eye, parallel to the lip. Intraorally the margins around the neoplastic lesion are measured and marked with a sterile marker. The labial and oral mucosa are incised along the preplanned line using a blade. Stay sutures, a skin hook, or retractors can be used to elevate the lip away from the surgical field. A periosteal elevator is used to dissect the gingival and labial mucosa away laterally and the palatine periosteum and mucosa medially until the bone is exposed along the entirety of the planned osteotomy line.

Atlas of Surgical Approaches to Soft Tissue and Oncologic Diseases in the Dog and Cat, First Edition. Marije Risselada.
© 2020 John Wiley & Sons, Inc. Published 2020 by John Wiley & Sons, Inc.

Combined Dorsolateral and Intraoral Approach to the Caudal Maxilla

I)

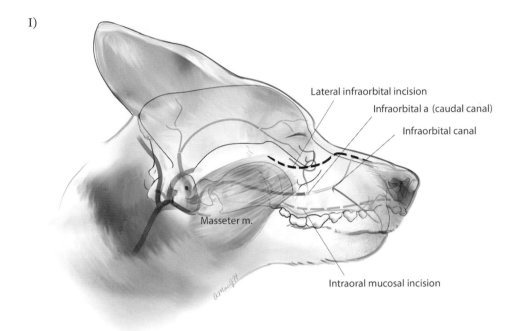

Lateral infraorbital incision

Infraorbital a (caudal canal)

Infraorbital canal

Masseter m.

Intraoral mucosal incision

II)

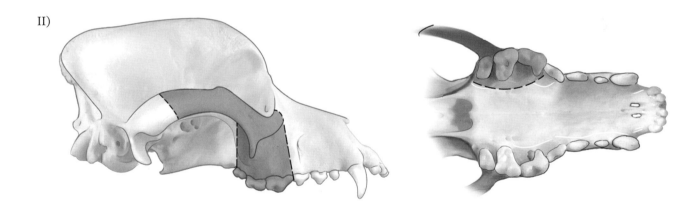

PATIENT POSITIONING AND DESCRIPTION OF THE PROCEDURE *continued*

III) The osteotomies can be performed with an osteotome and mallet, oscillating saw, high speed air drill, or a combination. The zygomatic arch osteotomy is performed first to allow access to the infraorbital artery. An ostectomy typically is necessary for exposure.

IV) The infraorbital artery is hemoclipped at its entry into the maxillary bone to minimize bleeding during the remainder of the osteotomies.

Combined Dorsolateral and Intraoral Approach to the Caudal Maxilla *continued*

III)

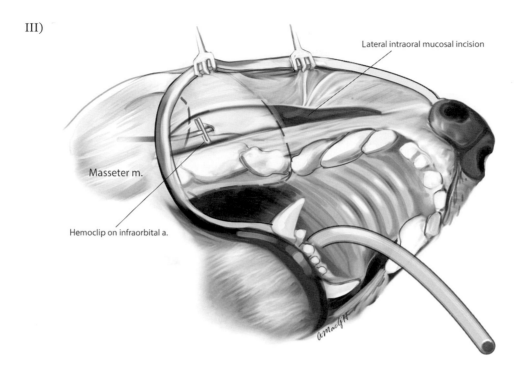

Lateral intraoral mucosal incision

Masseter m.

Hemoclip on infraorbital a.

IV)

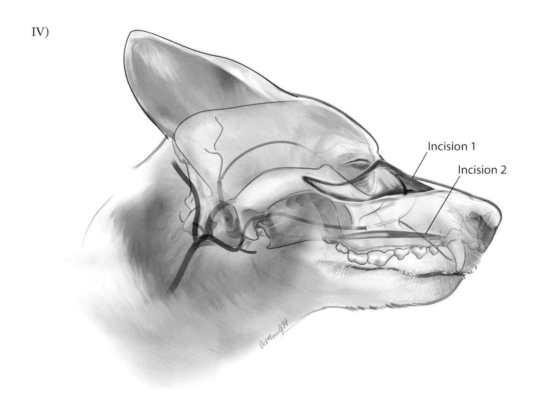

Incision 1

Incision 2

PATIENT POSITIONING AND DESCRIPTION OF THE PROCEDURE *continued*

V) The remainder of the osteotomies are performed to complete the ostectomy. With typically the lateral and dorsal aspects of the nasal bone first, then the palatine bone, leaving the caudal maxilla or medial orbit osteotomy for last.
  Turbinates are broken down by blunt and sharp dissection and the rostral maxilla removed. Bleeding from the hard palate and turbinates can be stopped by direct pressure, gauze soaked in cold saline, or hemostatic agents. If bleeding persists from the palatine artery, ligation or hemoclip application might be necessary.

CLOSURE

The skin incision is closed by first apposing the masseter muscle to the fibrous tissue ventral to the eye, after which the subcutaneous tissues and skin are closed routinely. The intraoral incision is closed in two layers: submucosa to the palatine periosteum and mucosa to mucosa. Bone tunnels can be drilled to anchor the submucosa to the palatine bone and periosteum if any tension is appreciated during closure. The mucosal closure can be a simple interrupted or a simple continuous closure pattern.

ALTERNATE POSITIONING AND APPROACHES

- In cases where extensive bleeding is expected a Rummel tourniquet can be preplaced around the ipsilateral external carotid artery, allowing it to be tightened if hemorrhage occurs during dissection.

Combined Dorsolateral and Intraoral Approach to the Caudal Maxilla *continued*

V)

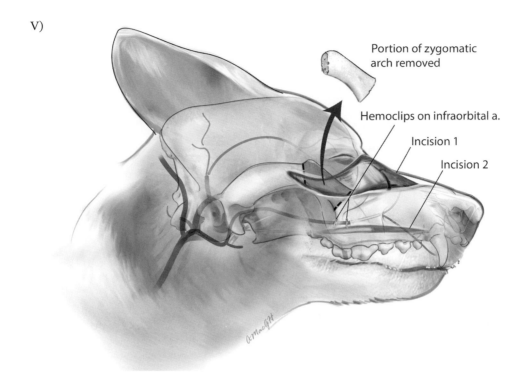

Portion of zygomatic arch removed

Hemoclips on infraorbital a.

Incision 1

Incision 2

Approach to the Zygomatic Arch[2,3]

INDICATIONS

- Zygomatic arch neoplasia
- Zygomatic sialoadenectomy
- Malunion of mandibular or zygomatic arch fractures

PATIENT POSITIONING AND DESCRIPTION OF THE PROCEDURE

I) The patient is placed in lateral recumbency with the forelimbs pulled caudally.

   The lateral area of the head, including the ear/pinna, and upper lip are clipped and aseptically prepared. The head is elevated on a sandbag/towel and the muzzle can be taped down to provide more stability.

II, III) The zygomatic arch is palpated and the incision is centered over the zygomatic arch, starting ventral to the lateral canthus and extending caudally over the temporomandibular joint. The platysma and sphincter colli profundus muscles are incised along the same line.

   The masseter muscles ventrally and the temporalis muscle caudodorsally are incised along the zygomatic arch and elevated off the bone using a periosteal elevator.

Atlas of Surgical Approaches to Soft Tissue and Oncologic Diseases in the Dog and Cat, First Edition. Marije Risselada.
© 2020 John Wiley & Sons, Inc. Published 2020 by John Wiley & Sons, Inc.

Approach to the Zygomatic Arch

I)

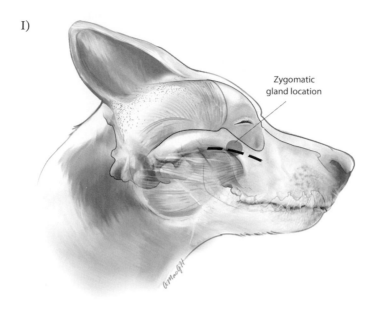

Zygomatic
gland location

II)

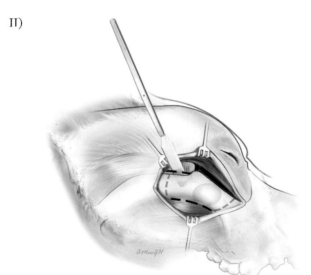

III)

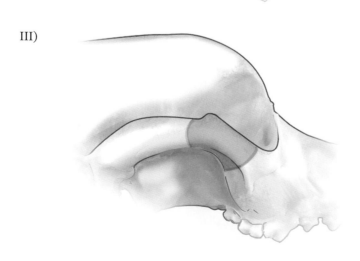

PATIENT POSITIONING AND DESCRIPTION OF THE PROCEDURE *continued*

IV) The muscular elevation is continued along the medial aspect, taking care not to damage the zygomatic salivary gland, to allow removal of the zygomatic arch.

CLOSURE

If the bone is replaced after sialoadenectomy, bone tunnels are drilled in the ostectomized bone and the bone rostral and caudal to the ostectomy site. The masseter muscle is sutured to the temporal muscle and its fascia. The superficial muscle layers, subcutaneous tissue, and skin are sutured in three layers.

ALTERNATE POSITIONING AND APPROACHES

- If a neoplastic lesion is resected en bloc with the zygomatic arch, the dissection can be wider dorsally and ventrally with a margin around the lesion.
- For a non-neoplastic disease of the salivary gland, the approach can be altered to lift the periosteum and fascia off the dorsal aspect of the zygomatic arch and retracting the periorbital fat dorsally. The access is enlarged by removing the dorsal aspect of the zygomatic arch with rongeurs.

Approach to the Zygomatic Arch *continued*

IV)

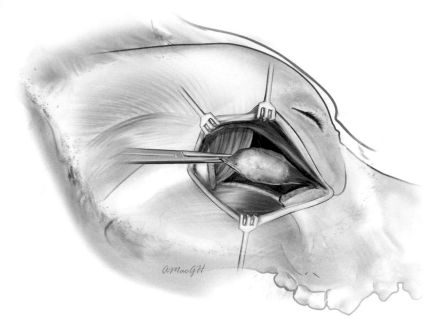

Approach to the Temporomandibular Joint[2]

INDICATIONS

- Condylectomy

PATIENT POSITIONING AND DESCRIPTION OF THE PROCEDURE

I)   The patient is placed in lateral recumbency with the forelimbs pulled caudally.
      The lateral area of the head, including the ear/pinna, and upper lip are clipped and aseptically prepared. The head is elevated on a sandbag/towel and the muzzle can be taped down to provide more stability.
      The zygomatic arch is palpated and the incision is centered over the caudoventral aspect of the zygomatic arch, starting over the center of the zygomatic arch and extending caudally over the temporomandibular joint.
II) The platysma and sphincter colli profundus muscles are incised along the same line. The caudal half of the masseter muscles inserting ventrally on the zygomatic arch are incised and elevated off the bone using periosteal elevators.

Atlas of Surgical Approaches to Soft Tissue and Oncologic Diseases in the Dog and Cat, First Edition. Marije Risselada.
© 2020 John Wiley & Sons, Inc. Published 2020 by John Wiley & Sons, Inc.

Approach to the Temporomandibular Joint

I)

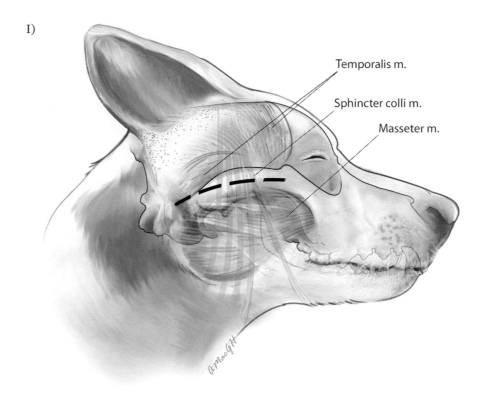

Temporalis m.

Sphincter colli m.

Masseter m.

II)

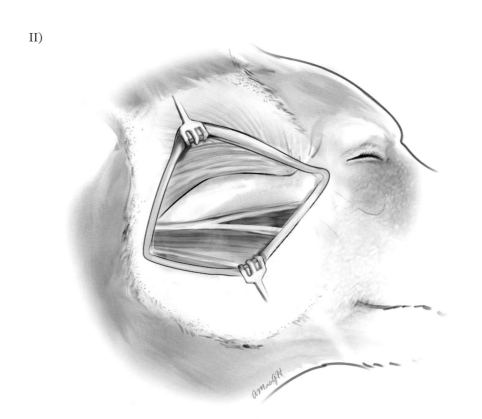

PATIENT POSITIONING AND DESCRIPTION OF THE PROCEDURE *continued*

III) The joint capsule will be visualized after elevation of the caudal aspect of the masseter muscles. The joint capsule is incised to access the temporomandibular joint.

CLOSURE

The joint capsule is closed first. The masseter muscle is sutured to the temporal muscle and its fascia. The superficial muscle layers, subcutaneous tissue, and skin are closed routinely in three layers.

Approach to the Temporomandibular Joint *continued*

III)

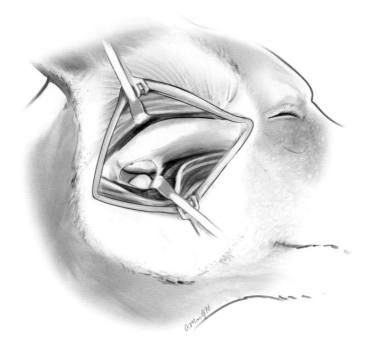

Dorsal Rhinotomy in the Dog[3,8]

INDICATIONS

- Access to the nasal cavity
- Intranasal biopsy or turbinate removal

PATIENT POSITIONING AND DESCRIPTION OF THE PROCEDURE

I) The patient is placed in ventral recumbency with the head elevated on a sandbag/towel and neck extended. The forelimbs can be flexed underneath and lateral to the thorax and next to the neck and head to allow for more stable positioning. Tape can be placed over the bridge of the nose to secure the head for the surgery.

   The dorsal skull and dorsal surface of the nose are clipped and aseptically prepared. The eyes should be palpable to allow for landmark identification. The planned incision line is indicated.

II) A midline skin incision is made from the level of the zygomatic process to the level of the edge of the nose. The periosteum is elevated off the bone and retracted. A tapered rectangular ostectomy is made with the smaller end towards the nose. The ostectomy cuts can be made with an oscillating saw, osteotome and mallet, or air drill.

CLOSURE

The bone does not need to be replaced. Closure is by approximating the periosteum and then the subcutaneous tissue in a simple continuous pattern, followed by routine skin closure.

ALTERNATE POSITIONING AND APPROACHES

- This approach can be extended dorsally to include a sinusotomy by combining this approach with the sinusotomy approach, using the landmarks for the sinusotomy to mark the dorsal extent.
- An alternate way to access the nasal turbinates and nasal cavity is through a ventral approach. The patient is placed in dorsal recumbency, with the oral cavity open. A midline incision is made through the mucosa and periosteum overlying the hard palate. A bone window is created to approach the nasal cavity. The mucoperiosteum and mucosa are closed in a single layer appositional pattern.

Atlas of Surgical Approaches to Soft Tissue and Oncologic Diseases in the Dog and Cat, First Edition. Marije Risselada.
© 2020 John Wiley & Sons, Inc. Published 2020 by John Wiley & Sons, Inc.

Dorsal Rhinotomy in the Dog

I)

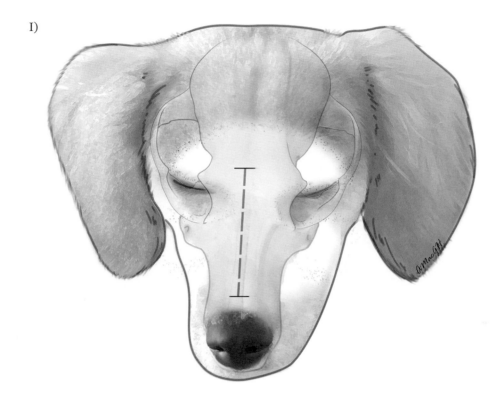

II)

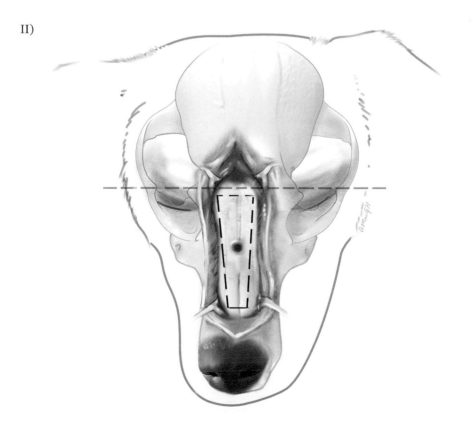

Dorsal Rhinotomy in the Cat[3,10]

INDICATIONS

- Access to the nasal cavity
- Intranasal biopsy or turbinate removal

PATIENT POSITIONING AND DESCRIPTION OF THE PROCEDURE

I) The dorsal skull and dorsal surface of the nose are clipped and aseptically prepared. The patient is placed in ventral recumbency with the head elevated on a sandbag/towel and neck extended. The forelimbs can be flexed underneath and lateral to the thorax and next to the head and neck to allow for more stable positioning. The eyes should be palpable to allow for landmark identification. The planned incision line is indicated.

II) A midline skin incision is made from the level of the zygomatic process to the level of the dorsal aspect of the nose. The periosteum is elevated off the bone and retracted. A tapered rectangular ostectomy is made with the smaller end towards the nose. The ostectomy cuts can be made with an oscillating saw, osteotome and mallet, or air drill.

CLOSURE

The bone does not need to be replaced. Closure is by approximating the periosteum and then the subcutaneous tissue in a simple continuous pattern, followed by routine skin closure.

ALTERNATE POSITIONING AND APPROACHES

- This approach can be extended dorsally to include a sinusotomy by combining this approach with the sinusotomy approach, using the landmarks for the sinusotomy to mark the dorsal extent.
- An alternate approach to the nasal turbinates is through a ventral approach. The patient is placed in dorsal recumbency, with the oral cavity open. A midline incision is made through the mucosa and periosteum overlying the hard palate. A bone window is created to approach the nasal cavity. The mucoperiosteum and mucosa are closed in a single layer appositional pattern.

Atlas of Surgical Approaches to Soft Tissue and Oncologic Diseases in the Dog and Cat, First Edition. Marije Risselada.
© 2020 John Wiley & Sons, Inc. Published 2020 by John Wiley & Sons, Inc.

Dorsal Rhinotomy in the Cat

I)

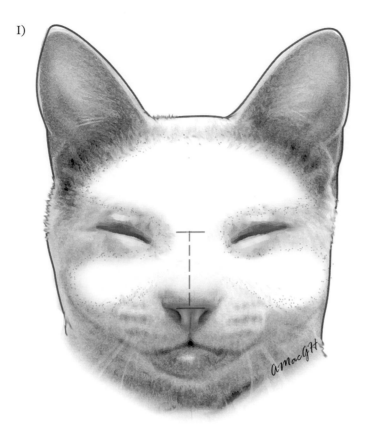

II)

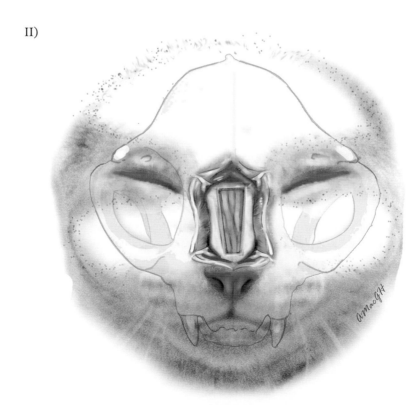

Dorsal Approach to the Sinuses in the Dog[3,8]

INDICATIONS

- Sinusotomy for biopsy
- Trephination

PATIENT POSITIONING AND DESCRIPTION OF THE PROCEDURE

I) The patient is placed in ventral/sternal recumbency with the head and neck elevated on a sandbag/towel. The forelimbs can be flexed underneath and lateral to the thorax and next to the head and neck to allow for more stable positioning. Tape can be placed over the bridge of the nose to secure the head for the surgery.

   The dorsal surface of the skull and the nose is clipped and aseptically prepared. The eyes should be palpable to allow for landmark identification. The planned incision line is indicated with a dashed line.

   A midline skin incision is made from the level of the zygomatic process (dorsally) to the level of the medial canthus ventrally. The location of the sinuses is equidistant from midline to the medial canthus in a left to right direction.

   Access to the sinus is obtained using a Steinman pin at the horizontal line connecting the zygomatic processes.

II) After obtaining access to the sinus with a Jacob's chuck, the sinusotomy can be enlarged with rongeurs. The bone does not need to be replaced.

CLOSURE

This is by approximating the deeper layers of subcutaneous tissue in a simple continuous pattern, followed by routine skin closure.

ALTERNATE POSITIONING AND APPROACHES

- Initial access to the sinus can either be at the level of the horizontal line connecting the zygomatic processes ('X') or in the middle (dorsoventral direction) between the horizontal lines connecting the zygomatic processes and the medial canthi ('●').
- Drains can be placed into the sinusotomy incisions/ostectomies and exited through a stab incision lateral to the initial approach to allow for postoperative flushing of the sinus.

Atlas of Surgical Approaches to Soft Tissue and Oncologic Diseases in the Dog and Cat, First Edition. Marije Risselada.
© 2020 John Wiley & Sons, Inc. Published 2020 by John Wiley & Sons, Inc.

Dorsal Approach to the Sinuses in the Dog

I)

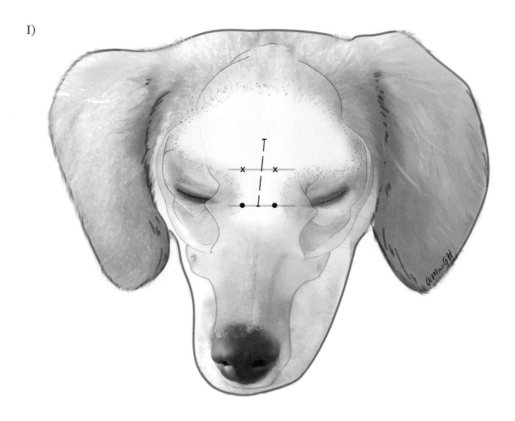

II)

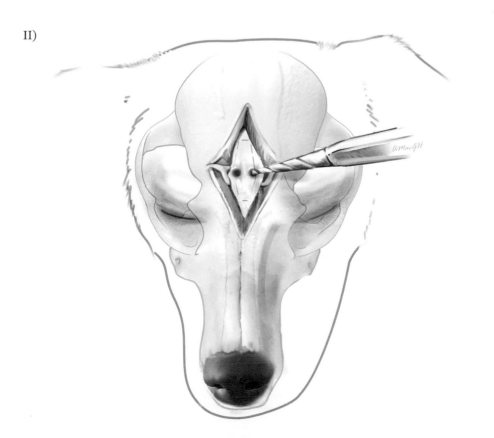

Dorsal Approach to the Sinuses in the Cat[3,10]

INDICATIONS

- Sinusotomy for biopsy
- Trephination

PATIENT POSITIONING AND DESCRIPTION OF THE PROCEDURE

I) The dorsal skull and dorsal surface of the nose are clipped and aseptically prepared. The patient is placed in ventral recumbency with the head elevated on a sandbag/towel and neck extended. The forelimbs can be flexed underneath and lateral to the thorax and next to the head and neck to allow for more stable positioning. The eyes should be palpable to allow for landmark identification. The planned incision line is indicated.

II) A midline skin incision is made from the level of the zygomatic process to the level of the medial canthus. An imaginary horizontal line is drawn at the level of the supraorbital processes or lateral canthi. The sinusotomy is made 0.5 cm from midline (either left or right) on this horizontal line.

   After obtaining access to the sinus with a Jacob's chuck, the sinusotomy can be enlarged with rongeurs.

CLOSURE

The bone does not need to be replaced. Closure is by approximating the deeper layers of subcutaneous tissue in a simple continuous pattern, followed by routine skin closure.

ALTERNATE POSITIONING AND APPROACHES

- The incision can be extended rostrally to include a dorsal rhinotomy if needed.

Atlas of Surgical Approaches to Soft Tissue and Oncologic Diseases in the Dog and Cat, First Edition. Marije Risselada.
© 2020 John Wiley & Sons, Inc. Published 2020 by John Wiley & Sons, Inc.

Dorsal Approach to the Sinuses in the Cat

I)

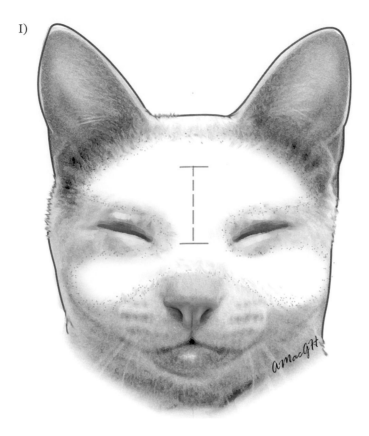

II)

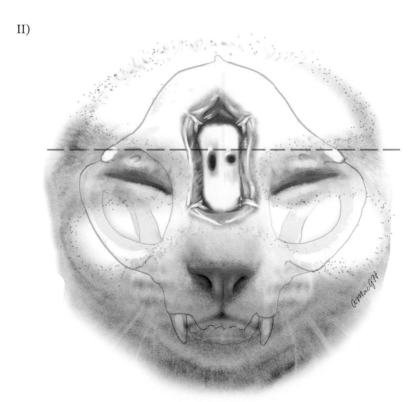

Section 2

Cervical Area and Ear

Approach to the Lateral Ear Canal[1,3]

INDICATIONS

- Lateral wall resection with or without ventral drain board
- Access to the ear canal

PATIENT POSITIONING AND DESCRIPTION OF THE PROCEDURE

I) The patient is placed in lateral recumbency with the forelimbs pulled caudally.

   The lateral area of the head, including the ear/pinna and upper lip, is clipped and aseptically prepared. The head is elevated on a sandbag/towel and the muzzle can be taped down to provide more stability. The skin incision depends on whether a drain board is planned. *No drain board*: a trapezoid-shaped skin incision is planned narrowing towards the ventral aspect and ending at the level of the horizontal canal. *With a drain board*: an hourglass-shaped incision with the narrowest part of the incision at the level of the horizontal canal – the ventral part of the hourglass is approximately half the length of the dorsal part.

II) The skin incision is made along the planned lines and the subcutaneous tissues and auricularis muscles (zygomatico-, cervico-, and parotidoauricularis) dissected away from the cartilage of the external ear canal. The parotid salivary gland is retracted ventrally to expose the junction between the vertical and horizontal canal.

Atlas of Surgical Approaches to Soft Tissue and Oncologic Diseases in the Dog and Cat, First Edition. Marije Risselada.
© 2020 John Wiley & Sons, Inc. Published 2020 by John Wiley & Sons, Inc.

Approach to the Lateral Ear Canal

I)

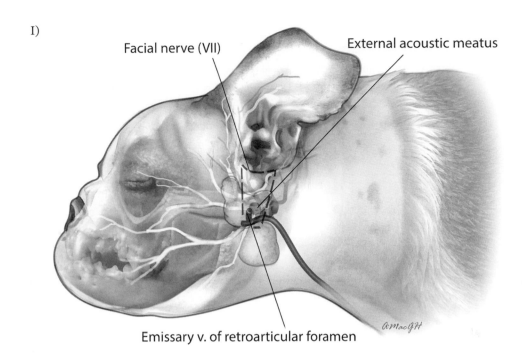

Facial nerve (VII)

External acoustic meatus

Emissary v. of retroarticular foramen

II)

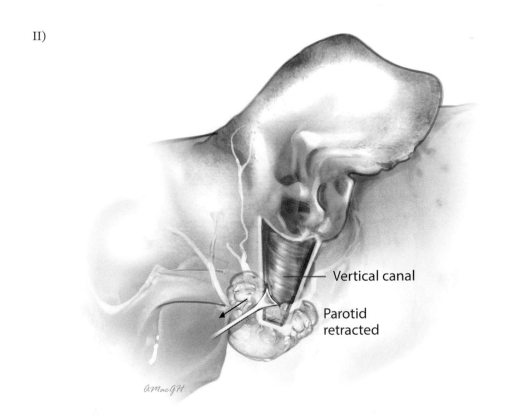

Vertical canal

Parotid retracted

PATIENT POSITIONING AND DESCRIPTION OF THE PROCEDURE *continued*

III) A full thickness incision through the cartilage is made at the cranial and caudal aspect, extending from the external opening of the vertical canal to the junction between the vertical and horizontal canal. Care is taken to leave 50–75% of the circumference of the canal to avoid cartilage necrosis, especially towards the ventral aspect.

IV) The cartilage flap is folded ventrally and trimmed to leave only 1–2 cm of drain board in place.

CLOSURE

This is achieved by mucosa to skin sutures, taking care to take a bite through the cartilage to ensure good purchase.

ALTERNATE POSITIONING AND APPROACHES

- A single linear incision over and parallel to the vertical canal can be used if only access to the ear canal is needed with a closure planned post surgery.
- *Subtotal ear canal ablation*: in this approach the initial circular incision is performed slightly lower, leaving more of the pinna, which allows for a slightly more unaltered ear carry. [11]

Approach to the Lateral Ear Canal *continued*

III)

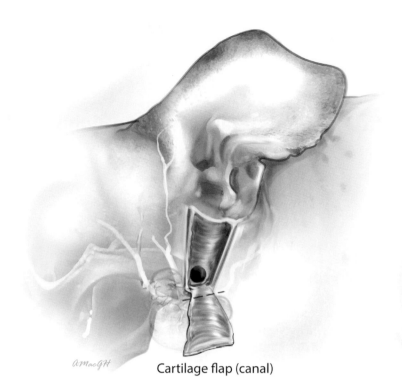

Cartilage flap (canal)

IV)

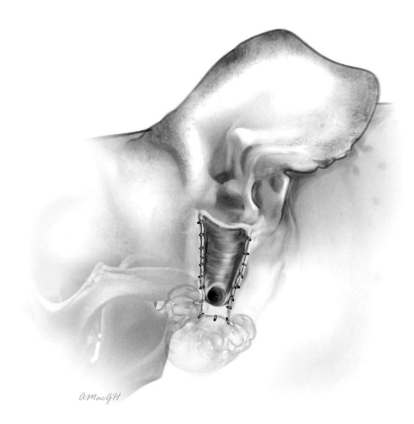

Approach to the Horizontal Ear Canal and Tympanic Bulla[3]

INDICATIONS

- Resection of vertical ear canal
- Total ear canal ablation with or without lateral bulla osteotomy

PATIENT POSITIONING AND DESCRIPTION OF THE PROCEDURE

I) The patient is placed in lateral recumbency with the forelimbs pulled caudally.

   The lateral area of the head, including the ear/pinna and upper lip, is clipped and aseptically prepared. The head is elevated on a sandbag/towel and the muzzle can be taped down to provide more stability. The skin incision is circular following the edges of the external opening of the vertical canal. Alternatively a vertical incision at the ventral edge of the circle can be added to extend the incision ventrally.

   A full thickness incision is made through the cartilage of the external ear canal along the planned circular line and the subcutaneous tissues and auricularis muscles (zygomatico-, cervico-, and parotidoauricularis) are dissected away from the cartilage of the external ear canal along with fibrous attachments. The parotid salivary gland is retracted ventrally to expose the junction between the vertical and horizontal canal.

II) The dissection is continued until the level of the bulla tympanica. Care is taken to identify and gently retract the facial nerve as it runs ventrally and slightly lateral to the horizontal canal. Once the horizontal canal is completely exposed, it is transected at the level of the bulla and the remaining attachments to the bulla removed.

Atlas of Surgical Approaches to Soft Tissue and Oncologic Diseases in the Dog and Cat, First Edition. Marije Risselada.
© 2020 John Wiley & Sons, Inc. Published 2020 by John Wiley & Sons, Inc.

Approach to the Horizontal Ear Canal and Tympanic Bulla

I)

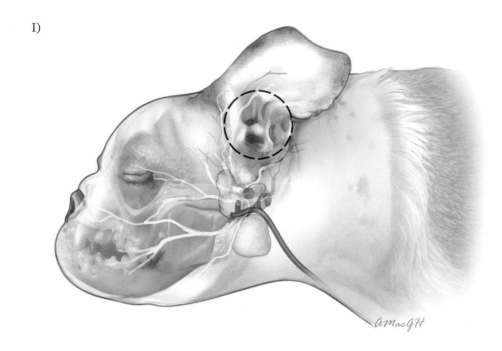

II)

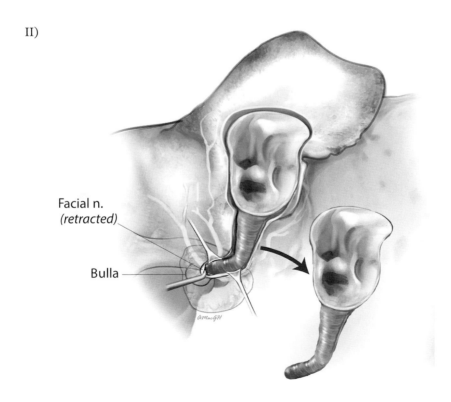

Facial n.
(retracted)

Bulla

PATIENT POSITIONING AND DESCRIPTION OF THE PROCEDURE *continued*

III) The external acoustic meatus is enlarged (bulla osteotomy) with rongeurs ventrally to allow a thorough curettage and lavage of the bulla. The craniodorsal aspect of the bulla (promontorium) is avoided to prevent damage to the semicircular canals or sympathetic nerves.

CLOSURE

The incision is closed primarily, apposing the deeper layers first, followed by subcutaneous and skin closure.

ALTERNATE POSITIONING AND APPROACHES

- *Subtotal ear canal ablation*: in this approach the initial circular incision is performed slightly lower, leaving more of the pinna, which allows for a slightly more unaltered ear carry. [11]

Approach to the Horizontal Ear Canal and Tympanic Bulla *continued*

III)

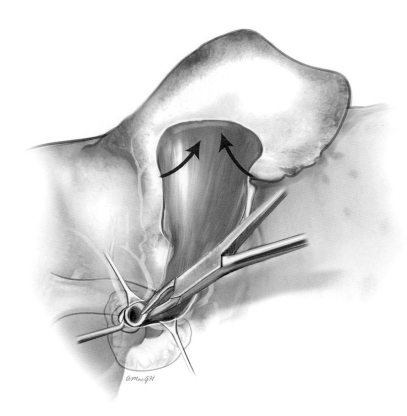

Ventral Approach to the Tympanic Bulla in the Dog[3]

INDICATIONS

- Access to the tympanic bulla
- Ventral bulla osteotomy (VBO)

PATIENT POSITIONING AND DESCRIPTION OF THE PROCEDURE

I) The patient is positioned in dorsal recumbency with the forelimbs pulled caudally. The area in between the mandibular rami and the cranial part of the neck is prepared for surgery. The neck is extended and elevated by placing a sandbag/towel underneath. The head can be taped down for increased stability. The larynx and horizontal rami of the mandible are palpated and serve as landmarks. A paramedian ventral incision is made between midline and the mandibular ramus on the affected side, at the caudal aspect of the mandibular horizontal ramus. The platysma is incised and the bulla is palpated, situated at the level of the bifurcation into the maxillary and facial vein (FV).

II) The dissection is continued bluntly by separating the caudal aspects of the digastricus (D) and mylohyoideus (MH) muscles first. The caudal part of the mylohyoideus can be elevated from its medial attachment.

Atlas of Surgical Approaches to Soft Tissue and Oncologic Diseases in the Dog and Cat, First Edition. Marije Risselada.
© 2020 John Wiley & Sons, Inc. Published 2020 by John Wiley & Sons, Inc.

Ventral Approach to the Tympanic Bulla in the Dog

I)

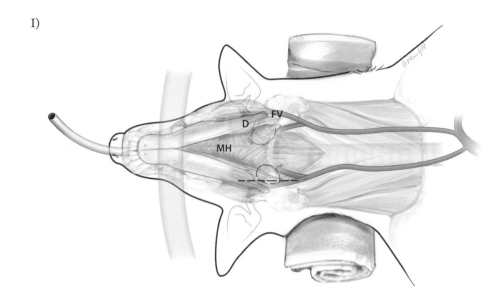

II)

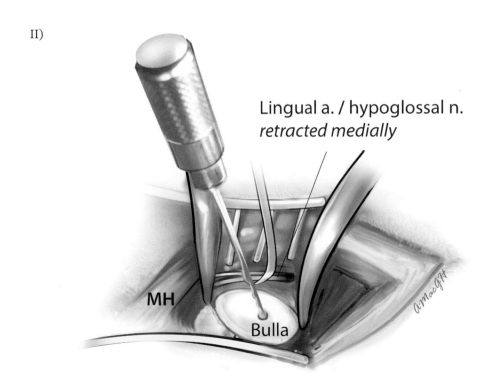

Lingual a. / hypoglossal n.
retracted medially

MH

Bulla

PATIENT POSITIONING AND DESCRIPTION OF THE PROCEDURE *continued*

III) The fibers of the hyopharyngeus muscle are deep to the first layer and are separated, taking care to carefully retract the hypoglossal nerve. The bulla is carefully cleaned from remaining fascial and muscle coverage with a periosteal elevator. The bulla is entered using a Steinman pin and opened up wider using rongeurs until the osteotomy site provides a large enough exposure.

CLOSURE

Wound closure is performed by reapposing the deeper layers and routine closure of the subcutaneous tissues and skin.

ALTERNATE POSITIONING AND APPROACHES

- For bilateral VBOs two paramedian incisions can be made or, alternatively, a longer midline incision.

Ventral Approach to the Tympanic Bulla in the Dog *continued*

III)

Lingual a. / hypoglossal n.
retracted medially

MH

Ventral Approach to the Tympanic Bulla in the Cat[3]

INDICATIONS

- Access to the tympanic bulla
- Ventral bulla osteotomy (VBO)

PATIENT POSITIONING AND DESCRIPTION OF THE PROCEDURE

I) The patient is positioned in dorsal recumbency with the forelimbs pulled caudally. The area in between the mandibular rami and the cranial part of the neck is prepared for surgery. The neck is extended and elevated by placing a sandbag/towel underneath. The head can be taped down for increased stability. The larynx and horizontal rami of the mandible are palpated and serve as landmarks.

II) A ventral incision is made between midline and the mandibular ramus on the affected side, at the caudal aspect of the mandibular horizontal ramus. The platysma is incised and the bulla is palpated, situated at the level of the bifurcation into the maxillary and facial vein. The dissection is continued bluntly by separating the caudal aspects of the digastricus (D) and mylohyoideus (MH) muscles first.

Atlas of Surgical Approaches to Soft Tissue and Oncologic Diseases in the Dog and Cat, First Edition. Marije Risselada.
© 2020 John Wiley & Sons, Inc. Published 2020 by John Wiley & Sons, Inc.

Ventral Approach to the Tympanic Bulla in the Cat

I)

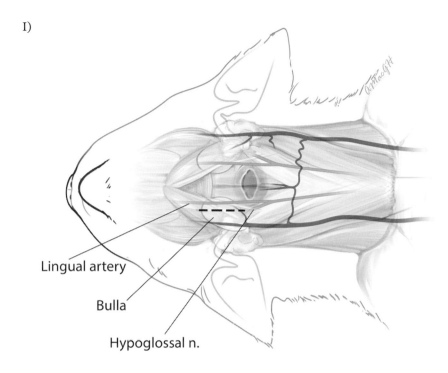

Lingual artery

Bulla

Hypoglossal n.

II)

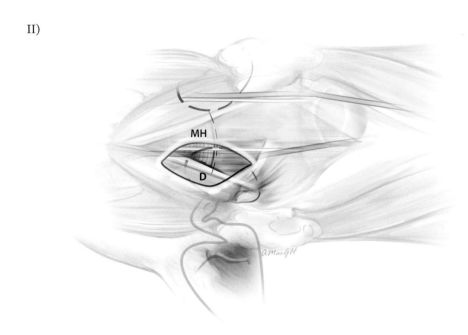

PATIENT POSITIONING AND DESCRIPTION OF THE PROCEDURE *continued*

III) The fibers of the hyopharyngeus muscle are deep to the first layer and are separated, taking care to carefully retract the hypoglossal nerve. The bulla is carefully cleaned from remaining fascial and muscle coverage with a periosteal elevator. The bulla is entered using a Steinman pin and opened up wider using rongeurs until the osteotomy site provides a large enough exposure.

IV) Care is taken to open up both compartments of the bulla (the dorsolateral and ventromedial chambers) in order to inspect and clean the entire bulla.

CLOSURE

Wound closure is performed by reapposing the deeper layers and routine closure of the subcutaneous tissues and skin.

ALTERNATE POSITIONING AND APPROACHES

- For bilateral VBOs two paramedian incisions can be made or, alternatively, a longer midline incision.

Ventral Approach to the Tympanic Bulla in the Cat *continued*

III)

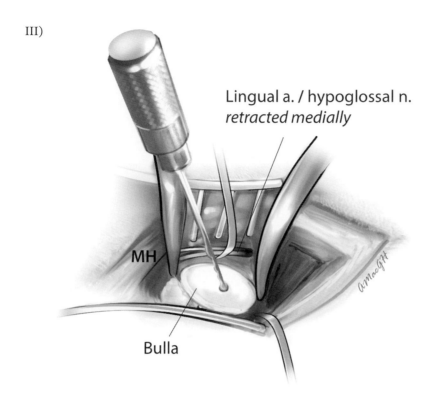

Lingual a. / hypoglossal n.
retracted medially

MH

Bulla

IV)

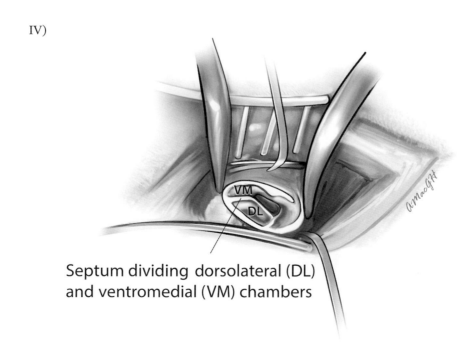

Septum dividing dorsolateral (DL)
and ventromedial (VM) chambers

Lateral Approach to the Mandibular and Sublingual Salivary Glands[3,12]

INDICATIONS

- Sialoadenectomy of the mandibular and sublingual salivary glands

PATIENT POSITIONING AND DESCRIPTION OF THE PROCEDURE

I) The patient is placed in lateral recumbency with the forelimbs pulled caudally.

   The lateral area of the head, including the ear/pinna, and upper lip, is clipped and aseptically prepared. The head is elevated on a sandbag/towel and the muzzle can be taped down to provide more stability. The mandibular salivary gland is situated at the bifurcation of the external jugular vein into the maxillary and linguofacial veins.

II) A longitudinal skin incision is made, centered over the mandibular salivary gland, extending from the bifurcation to the caudal edge of the mandible. The subcutaneous tissue, platysma, and parotidoauricularis muscles are bluntly dissected away to expose the capsule of the salivary gland.

   Dissection is continued cranially to encompass the sublingual salivary gland. If the rostral aspect cannot be safely reached with caudal traction, the salivary gland complex can be tunneled underneath the digastricus muscle to aid in better exposure or the digastricus muscle can be transected.[a]

---

[a] The digastricus muscle can be transected and reapposed to aid in better exposure if needed. Transection would occur along the dotted line (Figure II) and as shown in Figure III (for illustrative clarity).

Atlas of Surgical Approaches to Soft Tissue and Oncologic Diseases in the Dog and Cat, First Edition. Marije Risselada.
© 2020 John Wiley & Sons, Inc. Published 2020 by John Wiley & Sons, Inc.

Lateral Approach to the Mandibular and Sublingual Salivary Glands

I)

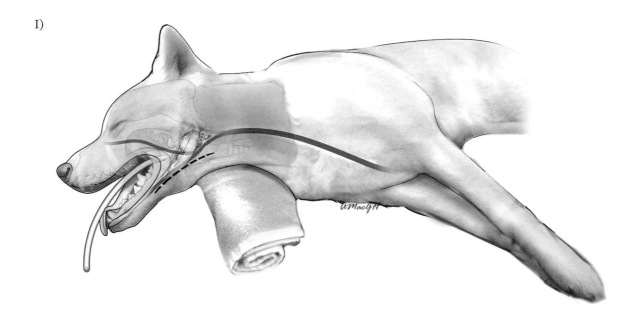

II)

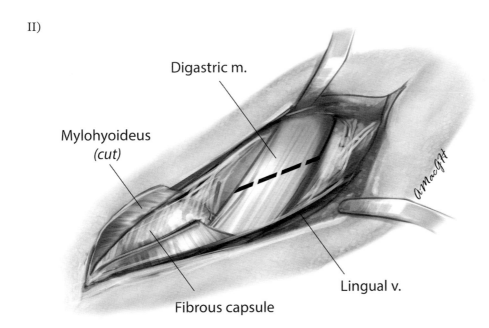

Digastric m.

Mylohyoideus
(cut)

Lingual v.

Fibrous capsule

PATIENT POSITIONING AND DESCRIPTION OF THE PROCEDURE *continued*

III) The bulk of the mandibular salivary gland (MG) gland is removed and the remainder is tunneled under the digastricus muscles to continue dissection cranially to remove the sublingual portion of the salivary gland complex. The can be done by placing a mosquito forceps on the duct or temporarily ligating the duct to use the suture tag as a stay suture. Craniomedial traction of the duct will allow further cranial dissection.

CLOSURE

This is by approximating the deeper tissues and routine closure of the subcutaneous tissues and skin.

ALTERNATE POSITIONING AND APPROACHES

- A ventral approach can be used, especially in bilaterally affected animals.

Lateral Approach to the Mandibular and Sublingual Salivary Glands *continued*

III)

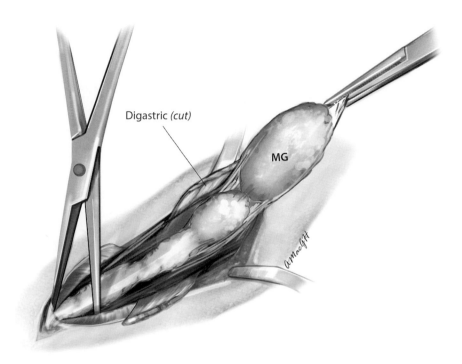

Digastric *(cut)*

MG

Ventral Approach to the Mandibular and Sublingual Salivary Glands[3,13]

INDICATIONS

- Uni- or bilateral mandibular sialoadenectomy
- Uni- or bilateral sublingual sialoadenectomy

PATIENT POSITIONING AND DESCRIPTION OF THE PROCEDURE

I) The patient is positioned in dorsal recumbency with the forelimbs pulled caudally. The area in between the mandibular rami and the cranial part of the neck is prepared for surgery. The neck is extended and elevated by placing a sandbag/towel underneath. The head can be taped down for increased stability. The larynx and horizontal rami of the mandible are palpated and serve as landmarks. A ventral incision is made between midline and the mandibular ramus on the affected side, at the caudal aspect of the mandibular horizontal ramus.

II) The subcutaneous tissues and platysma muscle are dissected to expose either the lymph nodes (MLN) or the salivary gland complex. The lymph nodes are located more laterally and superficial to the mandibular salivary gland (MG).

For a sialoadenectomy, the mandibular salivary gland (MG) is exposed first. Dissection is continued cranially along the sublingual salivary gland (SLG) to expose the digastricus muscle. The dissected salivary gland is tunneled underneath (dorsal to) the digastricus muscle and dissection continued cranially along the sublingual salivary gland.

CLOSURE

Wound closure is performed by reapposing the deeper layers and routine closure of the subcutaneous tissues and skin.

ALTERNATE POSITIONING AND APPROACHES

- A lateral approach can be used for unilateral sialoadenectomies.
- The digastricus muscle can be transected and reapposed to aid in better exposure if needed.

Atlas of Surgical Approaches to Soft Tissue and Oncologic Diseases in the Dog and Cat, First Edition. Marije Risselada.
© 2020 John Wiley & Sons, Inc. Published 2020 by John Wiley & Sons, Inc.

Ventral Approach to the Mandibular and Sublingual Salivary Glands

I)

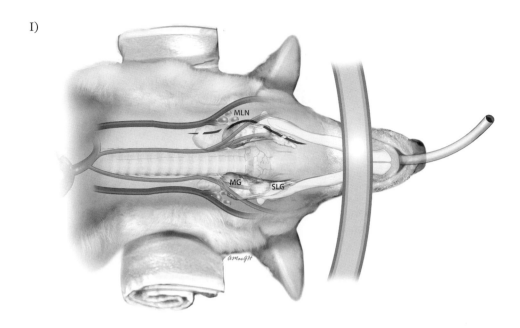

II)

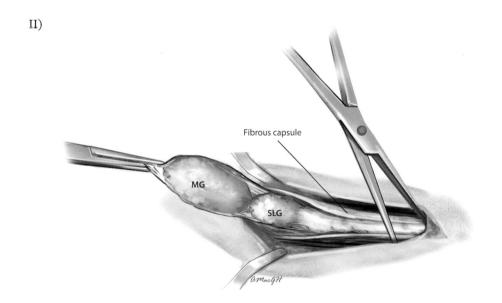

Lateral Approach to the Mandibular and Retropharyngeal Lymph Nodes[14]

INDICATIONS

- Unilateral mandibular lymph node removal
- Unilateral retropharyngeal lymph node removal

PATIENT POSITIONING AND DESCRIPTION OF THE PROCEDURE

I) The patient is positioned in lateral recumbency with the forelimbs pulled caudally. The lateral area of the head, including the ear/pinna and upper lip, is clipped and aseptically prepared. The neck is extended and elevated by placing a sandbag/towel underneath. The mandibular salivary gland is situated at the bifurcation of the external jugular vein (JV) into the maxillary and linguofacial veins.

II) A longitudinal skin incision is made, centered over the mandibular salivary gland, extending from the bifurcation to the caudal edge of the mandible. The subcutaneous tissue, platysma, and parotidoauricularis muscles are bluntly dissected away to expose the mandibular salivary gland. This gland is retracted laterally to expose the medial retropharyngeal lymph node (LN).

CLOSURE

Wound closure is performed by reapposing the muscles, followed by routine closure of the subcutaneous tissues and skin.

ALTERNATE POSITIONING AND APPROACHES

- A ventral midline approach can be used for bilateral lymph node removal. The ventral approach is more commonly used than the lateral as it allows for bilateral lymph node evaluation and removal.

Atlas of Surgical Approaches to Soft Tissue and Oncologic Diseases in the Dog and Cat, First Edition. Marije Risselada.
© 2020 John Wiley & Sons, Inc. Published 2020 by John Wiley & Sons, Inc.

Lateral Approach to the Mandibular and Retropharyngeal Lymph Nodes

I)

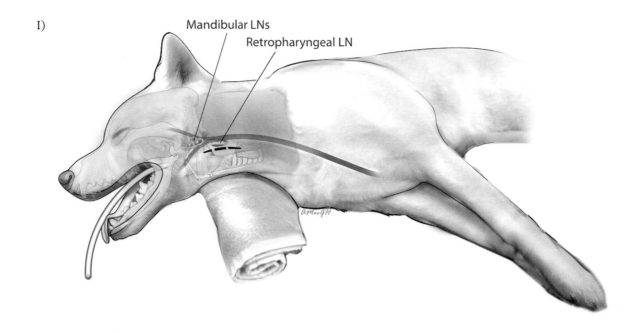

II)

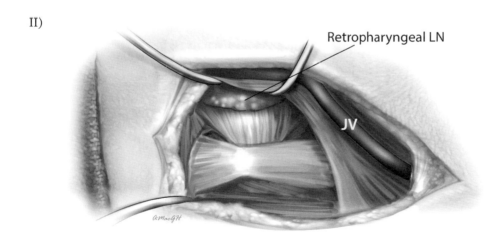

Ventral Approach to the Mandibular and Retropharyngeal Lymph Nodes[15]

INDICATIONS

- Mandibular lymphadenectomy
- Retropharyngeal lymphadenectomy

PATIENT POSITIONING AND DESCRIPTION OF THE PROCEDURE

I) The patient is positioned in dorsal recumbency with the forelimbs pulled caudally. The neck is clipped from the intermandibular area to the cranial thorax, extending dorsally along the lateral sides. The neck is extended and elevated by placing a sandbag/towel underneath. The head can be taped down for increased stability. The larynx and horizontal rami of the mandible are palpated and serve as landmarks. A ventral midline incision is made extending from the caudal third of the mandible cranially to the larynx caudally.

II) *Mandibular lymph node*: the subcutaneous tissues and platysma muscle are dissected to expose the mandibular lymph node (MLN) located at the caudal aspect of the horizontal ramus of the mandible with the facial vein over its ventral aspect.

Atlas of Surgical Approaches to Soft Tissue and Oncologic Diseases in the Dog and Cat, First Edition. Marije Risselada.
© 2020 John Wiley & Sons, Inc. Published 2020 by John Wiley & Sons, Inc.

Ventral Approach to the Mandibular and Retropharyngeal Lymph Nodes

I)

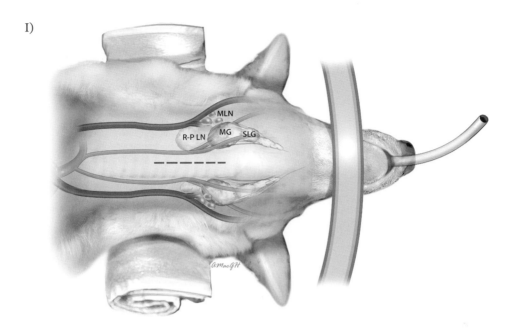

II)

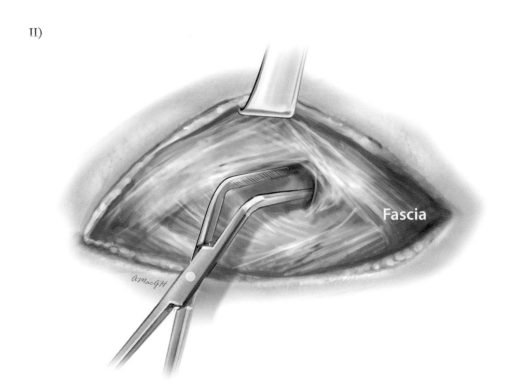

PATIENT POSITIONING AND DESCRIPTION OF THE PROCEDURE *continued*

III) *Retropharyngeal lymph node*: the lymph node (R-PLN) is visualized by identifying the mandibular salivary gland (MG) and the adjacent sublingual salivary gland (SLG) and retracting it laterally to expose the lymph node dorsally.

CLOSURE

Wound closure is performed by reapposing the deeper layers and routine closure of the subcutaneous tissues and skin.

ALTERNATE POSITIONING AND APPROACHES

- A lateral approach can be used for unilateral lymph node removal, potentially in conjunction with an orofacial tumor removal, without the need for repositioning.

Ventral Approach to the Mandibular and Retropharyngeal Lymph Nodes *continued*

III)

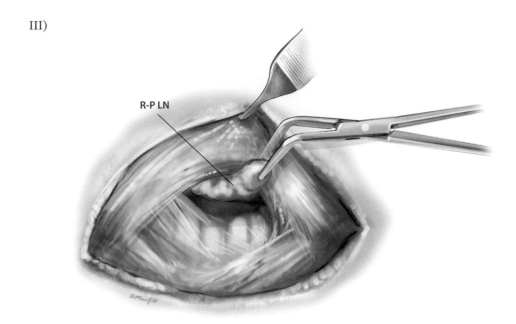

Lateral Approach to the Larynx[16]

INDICATIONS

- Arytenoid lateralization
- Cricopharyngeal myotomy/myectomy

PATIENT POSITIONING AND DESCRIPTION OF THE PROCEDURE

I) The patient is placed in lateral recumbency with the forelimbs pulled caudally.

The lateral area of the cervical area, from the mandible to the prescapular area, is clipped and aseptically prepared. The neck can be elevated on a sandbag/towel and slightly rolled/obliqued with the ventral aspect higher than the dorsal aspect if needed. The muzzle can be taped down to provide more stability.

II) A skin incision is made ventral to the jugular vein, and the jugular vein is lifted dorsally during blunt dissection. The platysma/sphincter colli muscle is divided and the deeper tissues are bluntly dissected while the jugular vein (JV) is retracted dorsally, until the thyroid cartilage can be grasped and the larynx rotated towards the surgeon. The thyropharyngeal (T-P) muscle is identified.

Atlas of Surgical Approaches to Soft Tissue and Oncologic Diseases in the Dog and Cat, First Edition. Marije Risselada.
© 2020 John Wiley & Sons, Inc. Published 2020 by John Wiley & Sons, Inc.

Lateral Approach to the Larynx

I)

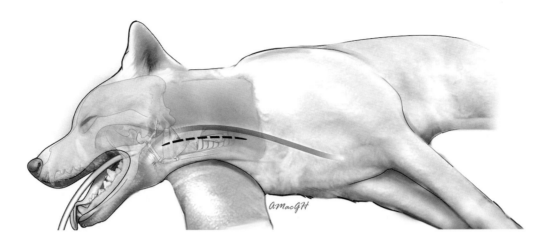

II)

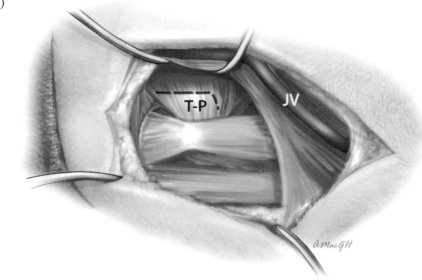

PATIENT POSITIONING AND DESCRIPTION OF THE PROCEDURE *continued*

III) Incise the thyropharyngeus muscle (T-P) along the caudodorsal edge of the thyroid cartilage. A stay suture or skin hook can be used to grasp the thyroid cartilage and retract ventrally. A fascial membrane is present deep to the thyropharyngeus muscle and is incised to gain access to the arythenoid and cricoid cartilages.

The cricoarytenoideus dorsalis muscle is identified and access to the cricoarytenoid joint is established by splitting the cricoarytenoideus dorsalis fibers mid-muscle (muscle splitting technique) or by transecting the muscle (classical technique). The transected cranial portion of the muscle can be used to aid exposure and access to the joint for suture placement.

CLOSURE

This is established by apposing the thyropharyngeus muscle first, followed by apposing the deeper tissues and then by routine closure.

ALTERNATE POSITIONING AND APPROACHES

- *Alternate techniques during the lateral approach*: splitting the thyropharyngeus muscle along its fibers rather than transecting.
- The cricoarytenoid joint is typically not disarticulated, but disarticulation will provide better exposure to the joint surface for suture placement if desired.
- An alternate approach to the larynx is a ventral midline approach.

Lateral Approach to the Larynx *continued*

III)

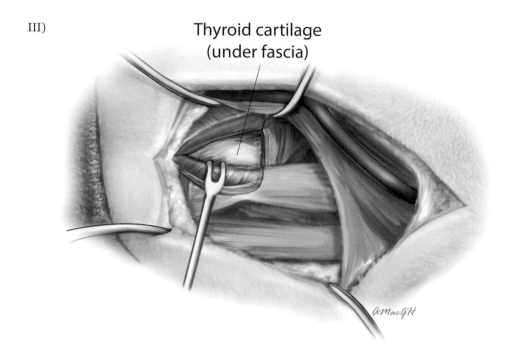

Thyroid cartilage
(under fascia)

Ventral Approach to the Larynx[1,3]

INDICATIONS

- Laryngotomy
- Laryngectomy
- Castellated laryngofissure

PATIENT POSITIONING AND DESCRIPTION OF THE PROCEDURE

I) The patient is positioned in dorsal recumbency with the forelimbs pulled caudally. The neck is extended and elevated by placing a sandbag/towel underneath. The maxilla can be taped down for increased stability while still allowing oropharyngeal access to the endotracheal tube. The larynx is palpated and a ventral midline incision from the hyoid apparatus to caudal to the larynx is made.

   The subcutaneous tissues and sphincter colli muscles are dissected to expose the paired sternohyoideus muscles. The sternohyoideus muscles are separated along the midline to access the thyroid and cricoid cartilages of the larynx.

II) *Laryngotomy*: a ventral midline laryngotomy is performed separating the paired thyroid cartilages using a blade to gain access to the laryngeal lumen.

Atlas of Surgical Approaches to Soft Tissue and Oncologic Diseases in the Dog and Cat, First Edition. Marije Risselada.
© 2020 John Wiley & Sons, Inc. Published 2020 by John Wiley & Sons, Inc.

Ventral Approach to the Larynx

I)

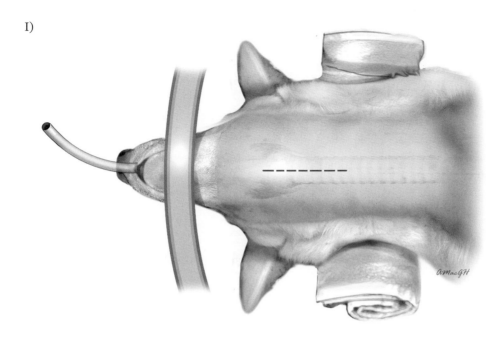

II)

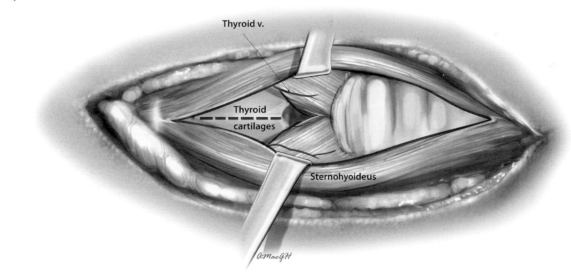

Thyroid v.

Thyroid cartilages

Sternohyoideus

PATIENT POSITIONING AND DESCRIPTION OF THE PROCEDURE *continued*

III) *Castellated laryngofissure*: the ventral midline incision in the thyroid cartilages follows the stepped incision line.

IV) *Castellated laryngofissure, continued*: the middle step is moved cranially and reattached to the cranial-most step, creating a larger luminal diameter.

CLOSURE

This is in two layers: the mucosa is closed in a simple continuous pattern using an absorbable suture, after which the thyroid cartilages are reapposed. Wound closure is performed by reapposing the sternohyoideus muscles, followed by routine closure of the subcutaneous tissues and skin.

ALTERNATE POSITIONING AND APPROACHES

- Arytenoid lateralization through a ventral approach has been described. This approach has the benefit of allowing access to both sides, but requires rotation of the larynx for access.

Ventral Approach to the Larynx *continued*

III)

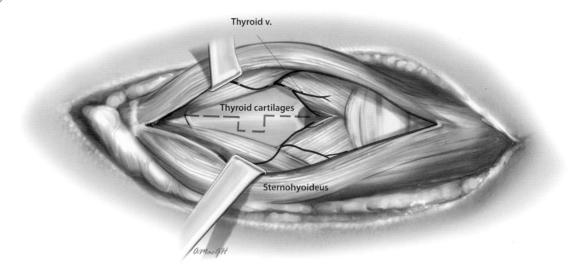

IV)

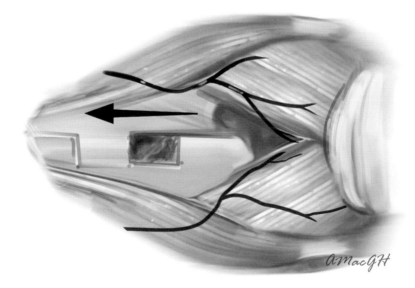

Ventral Approach to the Trachea, Esophagus, Carotid Sheath[1,3]

INDICATIONS

- Carotid artery ligation
- Tracheotomy
- Tracheal resection and anastomosis
- Esophagotomy

PATIENT POSITIONING AND DESCRIPTION OF THE PROCEDURE

I) The patient is positioned in dorsal recumbency with the forelimbs pulled caudally. The neck is clipped from the intermandibular area to the cranial thorax, extending dorsally along the lateral sides. The neck is extended and elevated by placing a towel/sandbag underneath. The maxilla can be taped down for increased stability while still allowing oropharyngeal access to the endotracheal tube. The larynx is palpated and a ventral midline incision made from the caudal aspect of the larynx to the manubrium.

II) The subcutaneous tissues and sphincter colli muscles are dissected to expose the paired sternohyoideus muscles. The sternohyoideus muscles are separated along midline to visualize the trachea and esophagus. The sternomastoideus muscles at the caudal aspect of the cervical area might need to be separated as well to allow access. Care is taken not to disrupt the blood supply to the thyroid glands towards the cranial extent of the incision.

    The trachea or esophagus are gently retracted and dissected bluntly to allow exposure for the respective tracheal or esophageal surgery.

Atlas of Surgical Approaches to Soft Tissue and Oncologic Diseases in the Dog and Cat, First Edition. Marije Risselada.
© 2020 John Wiley & Sons, Inc. Published 2020 by John Wiley & Sons, Inc.

Ventral Approach to the Trachea, Esophagus, Carotid Sheath

I)

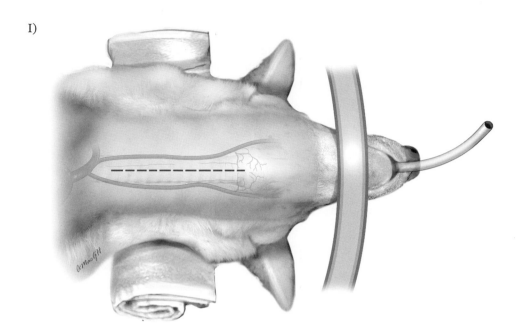

II)

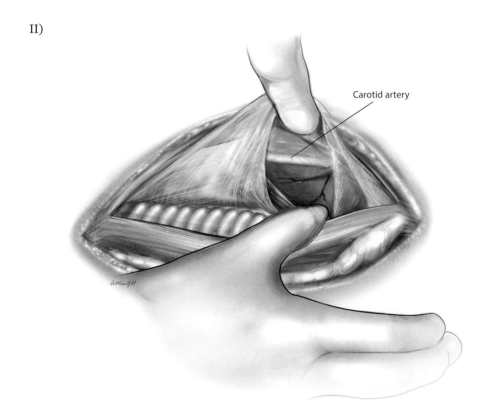

Carotid artery

PATIENT POSITIONING AND DESCRIPTION OF THE PROCEDURE *continued*

III) *Carotid artery ligation*: the trachea and esophagus are gently retracted away from the targeted carotid artery with either an army navy retractor or an assistant's finger. Blunt tipped self-retaining retractors could be used, such as Weitlaner or a baby Balfour, in the absence of an assisting surgeon. The carotid sheath is palpated, grasped with forceps, and opened to expose the neurovascular bundle within, making sure to identify the vagus and recurrent laryngeal nerves as well as the internal jugular. A single suture (silk or a non-absorbable monofilament, 2/0) is then passed around the carotid artery and tied.

CLOSURE

Wound closure is performed by reapposing the sternohyoideus muscles and the sternomastoideus muscles, followed by routine closure of the subcutaneous tissues and skin.

Ventral Approach to the Trachea, Esophagus, Carotid Sheath *continued*

III)

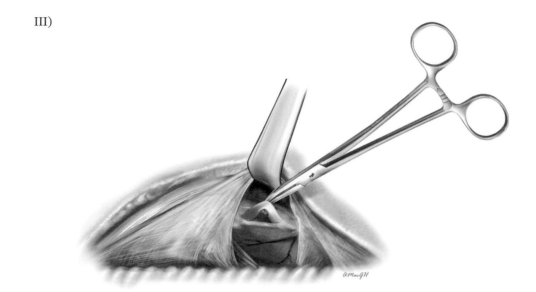

Ventral Approach to the (Para)Thyroid Glands[1,3]

INDICATIONS

- Uni- or bilateral thyroidectomy
- Access to all four parathyroid glands for parathyroidectomy

PATIENT POSITIONING AND DESCRIPTION OF THE PROCEDURE

I) The patient is positioned in dorsal recumbency with the forelimbs pulled caudally. The neck is clipped from the inter-mandibular area to the cranial thorax, extending dorsally along the lateral sides. The neck is extended and elevated by placing a sandbag/towel underneath. The maxilla can be taped down for increased stability while still allowing oropharyngeal access to the endotracheal tube. The larynx is palpated and a ventral midline incision made from the caudal aspect of the larynx to the mid- to caudal cervical area.

II) The subcutaneous tissues and sphincter colli muscles are dissected to expose the paired sternohyoideus muscles. The sternohyoideus muscles are separated along the midline to visualize the trachea and the thyroid glands, located at the level of the 5th–8th tracheal rings bilaterally. The external parathyroid is found at the cranial pole of the thyroid gland, and the internal parathyroid at the caudal pole.

   a) *Thyroidectomy*: the gland is dissected away from the surrounding tissues using a combination of blunt and sharp dissection and (electro)coagulation. The cranial and caudal thyroid vein and artery are ligated. The right common carotid artery, vagosympathetic trunk, and fibers of the right recurrent laryngeal nerve are in close proximity to the dorsal aspect of the right thyroid gland.

   b) *Parathyroidectomy*: the abnormal parathyroid gland is dissected away from the thyroid gland along with a cuff of normal thyroid tissue.

CLOSURE

Wound closure is performed by reapposing the sternohyoideus muscles, followed by routine closure of the subcutaneous tissues and skin.

Atlas of Surgical Approaches to Soft Tissue and Oncologic Diseases in the Dog and Cat, First Edition. Marije Risselada.
© 2020 John Wiley & Sons, Inc. Published 2020 by John Wiley & Sons, Inc.

Ventral Approach to the (Para)Thyroid Glands

I)

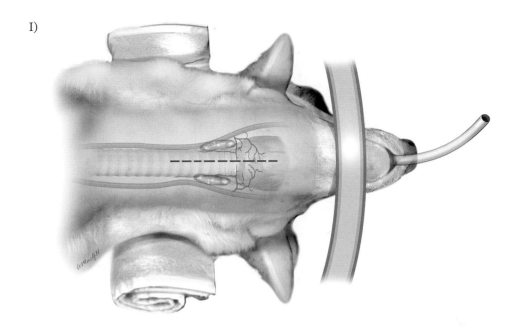

II)

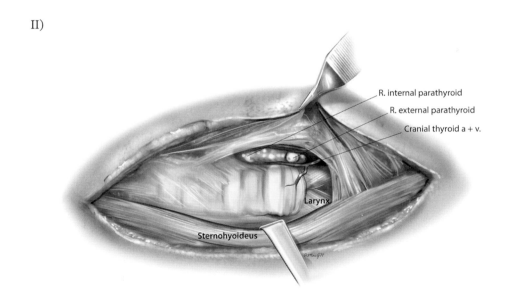

R. internal parathyroid
R. external parathyroid
Cranial thyroid a + v.
Larynx
Sternohyoideus

Approach to the Superficial Cervical Lymph Node[17]

INDICATIONS

- Lymph node biopsy or removal

PATIENT POSITIONING AND DESCRIPTION OF THE PROCEDURE

I) The patient is positioned in lateral recumbency with the neck extended and the forelimbs in a neutral position or pulled caudally. The lateral cervical area is clipped and prepped. If needed, a sandbag/towel can be placed under the neck to elevate the area away from the front leg. A skin incision is made cranial to the shoulder joint. The jugular vein (JV) is palpated and the skin incision planned dorsal to the vein.

II) The subcutaneous tissues and platysma muscle are dissected away to expose the omotransversarius (OM). The lymph node lies medial to the omotransversarius muscle and can be at either the dorsal or ventral aspect.

Atlas of Surgical Approaches to Soft Tissue and Oncologic Diseases in the Dog and Cat, First Edition. Marije Risselada.
© 2020 John Wiley & Sons, Inc. Published 2020 by John Wiley & Sons, Inc.

Approach to the Superficial Cervical Lymph Node

I)

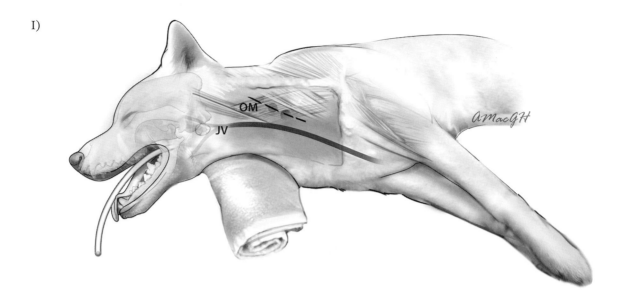

II)

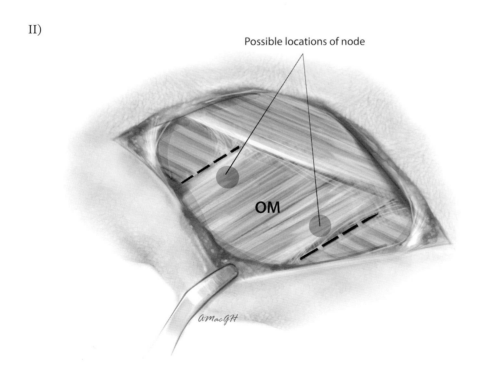

Possible locations of node

PATIENT POSITIONING AND DESCRIPTION OF THE PROCEDURE *continued*

III) The ventral or dorsal aspect of the muscle overlying the lymph node is bluntly dissected away from the surrounding tissue to allow retraction and exposure of the lymph node.

CLOSURE

Wound closure is routinely performed in multiple layers: the deep layer, reapposing the omotransversarius muscle, the deep subcutaneous tissue and platysma, and then a subcutaneous and skin layer.

ALTERNATE POSITIONING AND APPROACHES

- Alternative positioning of the patient is in dorsal or dorsolateral recumbency.[14]

Approach to the Superficial Cervical Lymph Node *continued*

III)

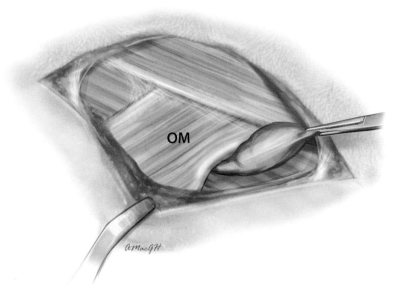

Section 3

Forelimb

Lateral Approach to the Scapula[2,17,18]

INDICATIONS

- Subtotal scapulectomy
- Total scapulectomy
- Approach to the scapular spine

PATIENT POSITIONING AND DESCRIPTION OF THE PROCEDURE

I, II) The patient is placed in lateral recumbency with the affected leg uppermost. The entire front leg, caudal cervical, and cranial thoracic areas – extending dorsal to the dorsal spinous processes – are clipped and prepped. The leg can be positioned and draped in a hanging limb position to allow draping of the lower leg and more maneuverability. A skin incision is planned along the spine of the scapula, extending dorsally to beyond the edge of the scapula.

Atlas of Surgical Approaches to Soft Tissue and Oncologic Diseases in the Dog and Cat, First Edition. Marije Risselada.
© 2020 John Wiley & Sons, Inc. Published 2020 by John Wiley & Sons, Inc.

Lateral Approach to the Scapula

I)

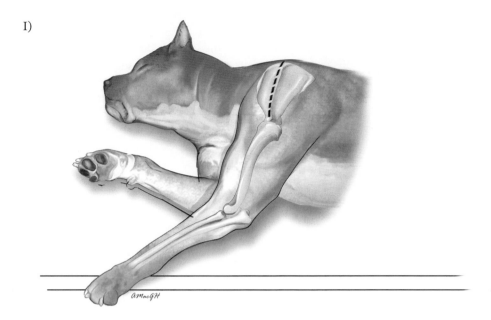

II)

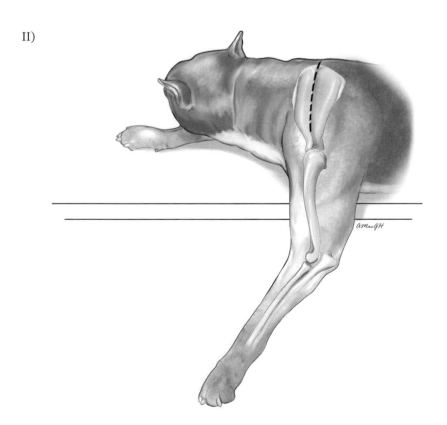

PATIENT POSITIONING AND DESCRIPTION OF THE PROCEDURE *continued*

III) The trapezius (Trap), omotransversarius (OM), and scapular portion of the deltoideus (Delt) muscles are incised (at an appropriate margin) and dissected away from the scapular spine.

IV) The supra- and infraspinatus muscles are dissected away from the scapular body to expose the anticipated area for the bone cut laterally. The serratus ventralis and rhomboideus muscles medially and the triceps (Tric) and teres major muscle caudally are dissected away from the scapular body, allowing lateral retraction and protection of the tissues medially during the osteotomy. The osteotomy can be performed with an oscillating saw, osteotome and mallet, or air drill.

CLOSURE

After removal of the scapula, the muscles are apposed to close the deeper layer and dead space in one or two layers. The overlying subcutaneous tissues are closed routinely.

ALTERNATE POSITIONING AND APPROACHES

- A soaker catheter can be placed in the defect prior to closure to aid in postoperative analgesia.
- Bone tunnels can be drilled in the remaining part of the scapula, large enough for large size non-absorbable sutures. These can be anchored in the deeper tissues or around the ribs if additional stability postoperatively is desired.
- The skin incision can be altered or planned around a mass if needed for oncologic purposes. Similarly, the site of the osteotomy is planned depending on oncologic margins.

Lateral Approach to the Scapula *continued*

III)

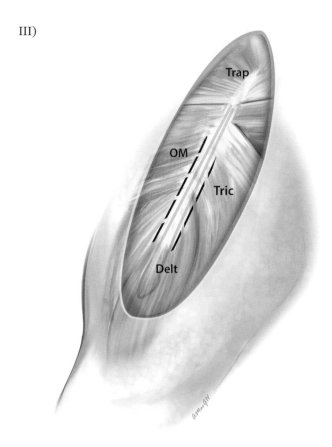

IV)

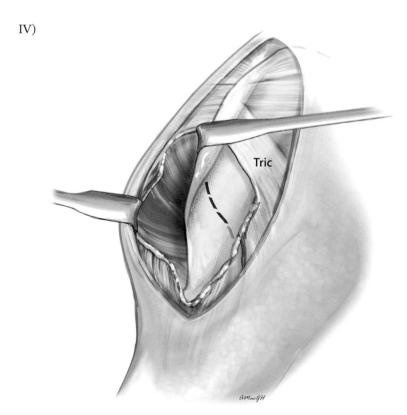

Dorsal Approach to the Spinous Processes and Scapula[2]

INDICATIONS

- Interscapular lesions
- Lesions of the cranial thoracic spinal processes

PATIENT POSITIONING AND DESCRIPTION OF THE PROCEDURE

I) The dorsal cervical and thoracic areas are clipped – extending bilaterally down the chest and neck. The patient is placed in sternal recumbency with the forelimbs flexed at the shoulders and elbows with the feet pointing forward.

 The skin incision is planned around the mass and extended far enough cranially and caudally to allow exposure to both scapulae. The subcutaneous tissue is bluntly dissected to expose the trapezius muscle.

 The omotransversarius (Omo) and latissimus dorsi (Lat) are shown for orientation.

II) The trapezius (Trap) muscle is incised away from the area to expose the rhomboideus (R) and serratus dorsalis (SD) muscles.

CLOSURE

The muscles are apposed to close the deeper layer and dead space in one or two layers. The overlying subcutaneous tissues are closed routinely.

ALTERNATE POSITIONING AND APPROACHES

- The patient can be tilted if access to only one scapula is desired.
- The forelimbs can be positioned with the elbows under the patient and the antebrachii internally rotated and pulled laterally to allow wider access to the spinous processes.
- If a partial scapulectomy is to be performed through this approach, the muscles are transected at an appropriate distance away from the bone and the planned ostectomy site is dissected free medially and laterally. If desired, bone tunnels can be drilled in the remaining part of the scapula, large enough for large size non-absorbable sutures. These can be anchored in the deeper tissues or around the ribs if additional stability postoperatively is desired. An alternative approach for a partial scapulectomy is through a lateral incision.

Atlas of Surgical Approaches to Soft Tissue and Oncologic Diseases in the Dog and Cat, First Edition. Marije Risselada.
© 2020 John Wiley & Sons, Inc. Published 2020 by John Wiley & Sons, Inc.

Dorsal Approach to the Spinous Processes and Scapula

I)

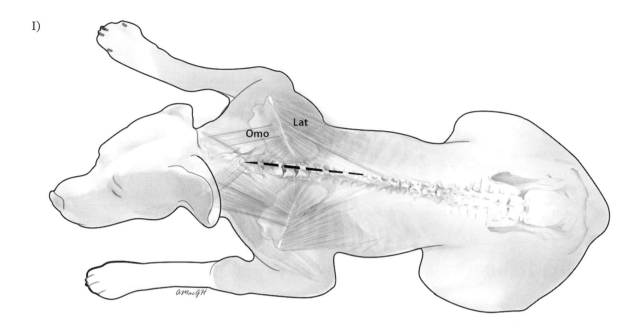

II)

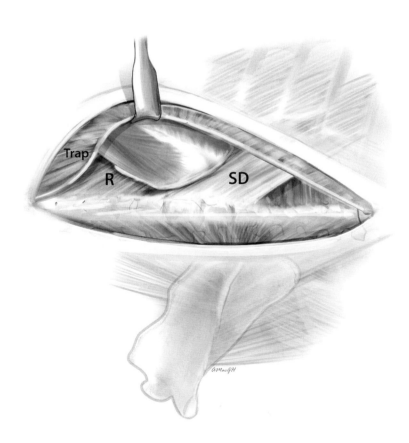

Forequarter Amputation: Lateral Approach[1,3,8,10,17]

INDICATIONS

- Non-salvageable forelimb lesions

PATIENT POSITIONING AND DESCRIPTION OF THE PROCEDURE

Ia,b)   The entire front leg, caudal cervical, and cranial thoracic areas – extending dorsal to the dorsal spines – are clipped and prepped. The patient is placed in lateral recumbency with the entire forelimb draped in and in a relaxed neutral position. A teardrop-shaped incision is planned along the scapular spine and around the forelimb at mid-humerus.

  II)   The subcutaneous tissues are bluntly dissected away to expose the trapezius (TR) muscles overlying the scapula and the omotransversarius (OM) muscle at the cranioventral aspect and the latissimus dorsi (LD) muscle caudally. The trapezius muscle is transected at the level of the scapula, exposing the rhomboideus muscle. The omotransversarius muscle is similarly transected. The latissimus dorsi muscle can be transected at this point or can be transected after elevating the scapula. Lateral retraction can be aided by placing a bone forceps on the scapular spine.

   The deltoideus and pectoral (Pec) muscles are shown for orientation.

Atlas of Surgical Approaches to Soft Tissue and Oncologic Diseases in the Dog and Cat, First Edition. Marije Risselada.
© 2020 John Wiley & Sons, Inc. Published 2020 by John Wiley & Sons, Inc.

Forequarter Amputation: Lateral Approach

I)

(a)   (b)

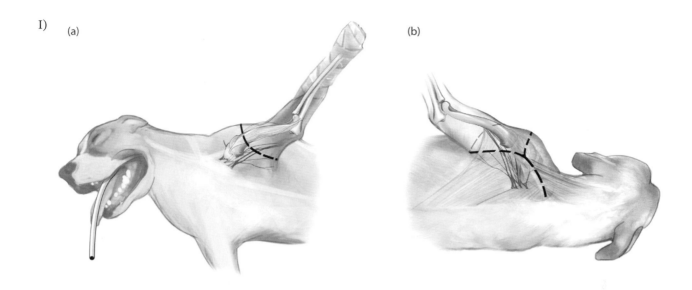

II)

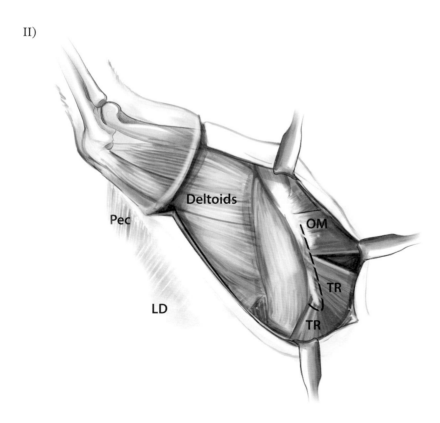

PATIENT POSITIONING AND DESCRIPTION OF THE PROCEDURE *continued*

III) The dorsal aspect of the scapula is retracted laterally to increase exposure to the rhomboideus (Rhomb, Rh) muscle, which is transected at its attachment on the scapula along with the serratus ventralis muscle. If not already performed, the latissimus dorsi muscle is transected at this point, freeing up the scapula.

IV) The brachial plexus, axillary artery, and axillary vein are bluntly dissected, double ligated, and transected while an assistant retains lateral retraction of the scapula. The superficial and deep pectoral muscles are transected along with any remaining attachments ventrally.

Forequarter Amputation: Lateral Approach *continued*

III)

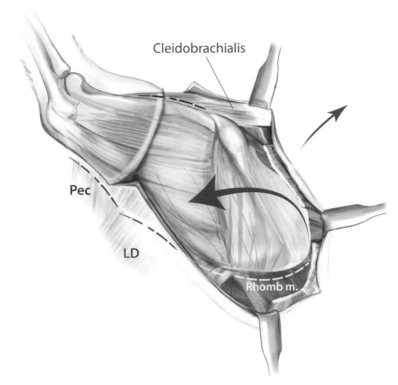

IV)

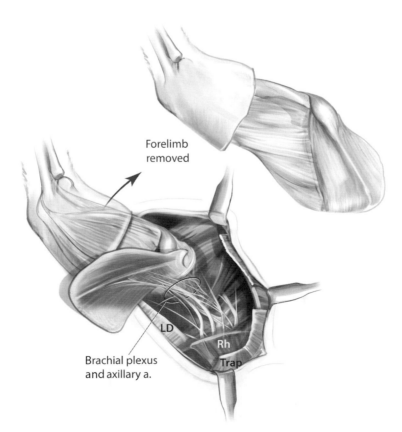

CLOSURE

V) Closure is by suturing the pectoral muscles dorsally overlying and protecting the exposed axillary artery, axillary vein, and brachial plexus, and layering the transected muscles to close the dead space and protect the ribs. The remainder of the closure is routine.

ALTERNATE POSITIONING AND APPROACHES

- While dissecting dorsally and medially, access might be facilitated with the surgeon positioned dorsal to the patient.
- *Alternative approach*: glenohumeral disarticulation for distal lesions.

Forequarter Amputation: Lateral Approach *continued*

V)

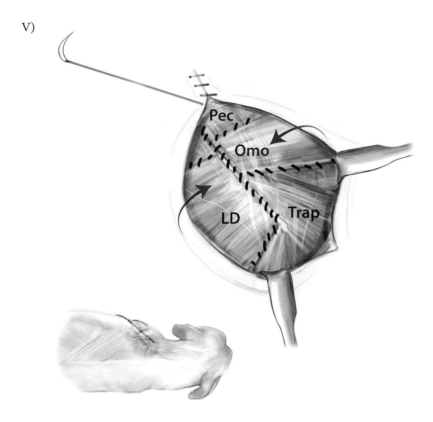

Ventral Approach to the Brachial Plexus and Axillary Artery[2,17]

INDICATIONS

- Brachial plexus tumor excision or biopsy
- Axillary artery ligation

PATIENT POSITIONING AND DESCRIPTION OF THE PROCEDURE

I) The patient is placed in lateral recumbency with the affected leg uppermost and retracted dorsally in abduction. The entire forelimb is prepped and draped. A semicircular skin incision is planned in the axilla.

II) The subcutaneous tissues are bluntly dissected away to expose the superficial (SP) and deep pectoral muscles, which are transected. A stay suture can be placed in the muscle ends to allow easier reappositioning and orientation. The latissimus dorsi muscle is retracted dorsally.

   The cleidobrachialis (CB) muscle is shown for orientation.

Atlas of Surgical Approaches to Soft Tissue and Oncologic Diseases in the Dog and Cat, First Edition. Marije Risselada.
© 2020 John Wiley & Sons, Inc. Published 2020 by John Wiley & Sons, Inc.

Ventral Approach to the Brachial Plexus and Axillary Artery

I)

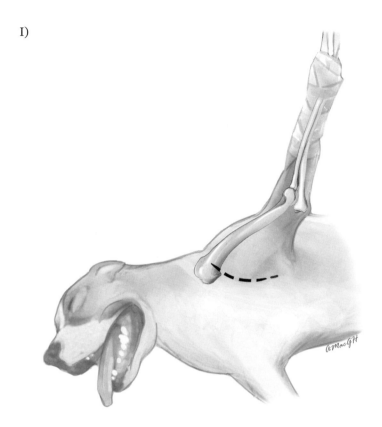

II)

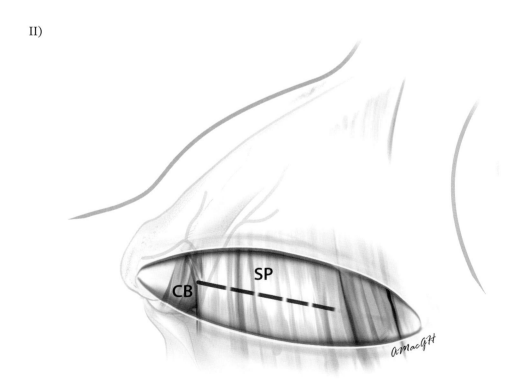

PATIENT POSITIONING AND DESCRIPTION OF THE PROCEDURE *continued*

III) The subscapularis (SubS) muscle and medial head of the triceps muscle (TM) are exposed and retracted to access the brachial plexus.

CLOSURE

The superficial and deep pectoral muscles (transected during the approach) are reanastomosed, while muscles that were separated and retracted during the approach are apposed. The remainder of the incision (subcutaneous tissue and skin) is closed routinely.

ALTERNATE POSITIONING AND APPROACHES

- An alternate approach to the brachial plexus is from a craniolateral direction.

Ventral Approach to the Brachial Plexus and Axillary Artery *continued*

III)

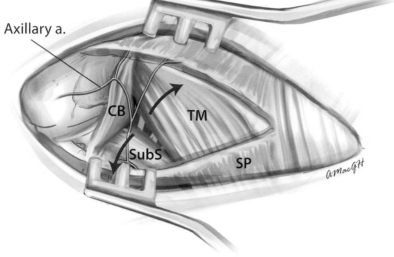

Craniolateral Approach to the Brachial Plexus[19]

INDICATIONS

- Brachial plexus tumor excision or biopsy

PATIENT POSITIONING AND DESCRIPTION OF THE PROCEDURE

I) The entire front leg and caudal cervical area are clipped and prepped. The patient is placed in lateral recumbency with the affected leg uppermost and in a relaxed neutral position (shown in a hanging limb prep position). A curved skin incision is planned at the cranial aspect of the shoulder joint, extending from mid-scapula to the proximal humerus. The subcutaneous tissues are bluntly dissected to expose the omotransversarius muscle.

II) The omotransversarius (Om) muscle is isolated and transected to allow lateral elevation of the cranial aspect of the scapula. The cranial extent of the transected muscle and the superficial cervical lymph node are retracted cranially, exposing the brachial plexus.

     The deltoideus (Delt) and trapezius (Trap) muscles are shown for orientation.

Atlas of Surgical Approaches to Soft Tissue and Oncologic Diseases in the Dog and Cat, First Edition. Marije Risselada.
© 2020 John Wiley & Sons, Inc. Published 2020 by John Wiley & Sons, Inc.

Craniolateral Approach to the Brachial Plexus

I)

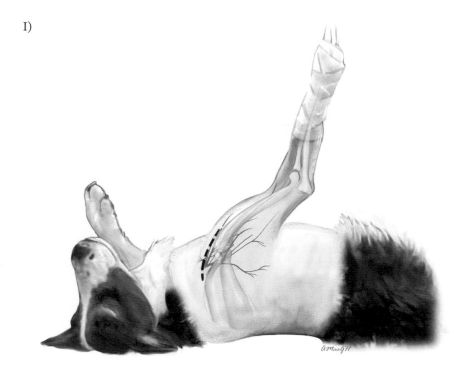

II)

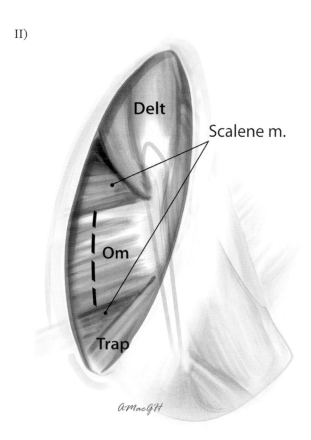

PATIENT POSITIONING AND DESCRIPTION OF THE PROCEDURE *continued*

III) The scalenus (Scal) muscle might have to be transected to allow exposure of the ventral branches of the C7, C8, and T1 nerves.

CLOSURE

The scalenus muscle, if transected, is reanastomosed first, followed by the omotransversarius muscle. Muscles that were separated and retracted are apposed, as are the deeper layers of the approach. The remainder of the incision (subcutaneous tissue and skin) is closed routinely.

ALTERNATE POSITIONING AND APPROACHES

- An alternative to this approach is a ventral approach to the brachial plexus.
- The leg can be positioned either in a hanging limb position during the surgery or in a relaxed neutral (non-hanging position).

Craniolateral Approach to the Brachial Plexus *continued*

III)

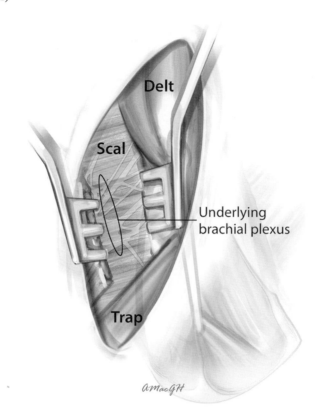

Section 4

Hindlimb

Partial/Middle Hemipelvectomy (Acetabulectomy)[20-22]

INDICATIONS

- Tumors localized to the acetabulum
- The cranial and caudal margin can be combined with the caudal margin and cranial margin of the total hemipelvectomy (a) to create a caudal hemipelvectomy (c) and cranial hemipelvectomy (not shown), respectively.

PATIENT POSITIONING AND DESCRIPTION OF THE PROCEDURE

I) The affected hindlimb, caudal abdomen, and lumbar area (extending to the contralateral side of midline) are clipped and prepped. The patient is placed in lateral recumbency with the affected leg uppermost in a hanging limb drape. The entire dorsal portion of the pelvis and caudal abdomen are draped in, allowing access circumferentially around the pelvis.

   The following structures are shown for orientation: semitendinosus (St), biceps femoris (BF), middle gluteal (MG), tensor fascia lata (TFL), sartorius (Sar), and epaxial (Epax) muscles and the sciatic (Sc) nerve. The ischium and ilium are similarly indicated.

Atlas of Surgical Approaches to Soft Tissue and Oncologic Diseases in the Dog and Cat, First Edition. Marije Risselada.
© 2020 John Wiley & Sons, Inc. Published 2020 by John Wiley & Sons, Inc.

Partial/Middle Hemipelvectomy (Acetabulectomy)

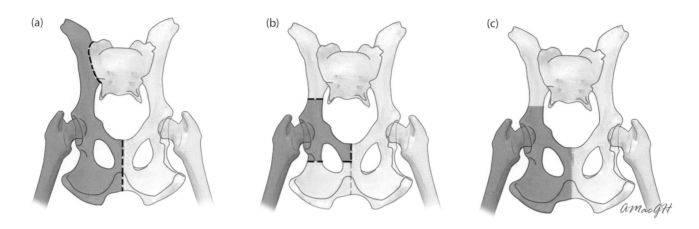

(a) (b) (c)

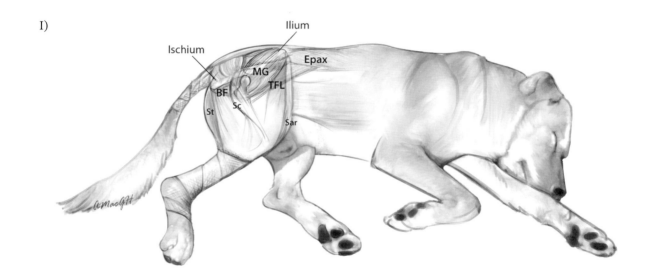

I)

PATIENT POSITIONING AND DESCRIPTION OF THE PROCEDURE *continued*

II, III) The incision line is planned along the dorsolateral aspect of the hip and along the inguinal canal, ensuring enough skin dorsolaterally to close the defect without tension.

Partial/Middle Hemipelvectomy (Acetabulectomy) *continued*

II)

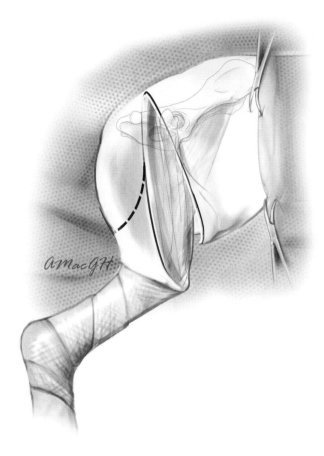

III)

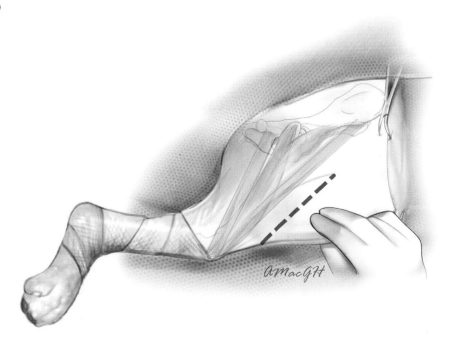

PATIENT POSITIONING AND DESCRIPTION OF THE PROCEDURE *continued*

IV) *Ventral dissection*: the subcutaneous tissues are dissected away from the midline to expose the medial thigh muscles (adductor, gracilis, and pectineus muscles). These muscles are elevated off the bone to expose the midline of the pubis with sufficient exposure for a pubic symphysiotomy. If desired, the symphysis can be left intact and osteotomies of the pubic and ischiatic bone can be performed closer to the ipsilateral side.

   The insertions of the abdominal muscles are similarly elevated off the bone. After the osteotomy, the intrapelvic muscles are carefully elevated off the bone medially.

V) *Dorsal dissection*: the skin is elevated to expose the biceps femoris (Bf), gluteal, and sartorial (Sar) muscles. The biceps femoris muscle is transected proximally and the gluteus muscles are transected at their insertion (middle, MG) or origin (superficial, SG). The deep gluteal muscle and piriform muscles are similarly transected.

   The following other structures are shown for orientation: semitendinosus (St) and tensor fascia lata (Tfl).

Partial/Middle Hemipelvectomy (Acetabulectomy) *continued*

IV)

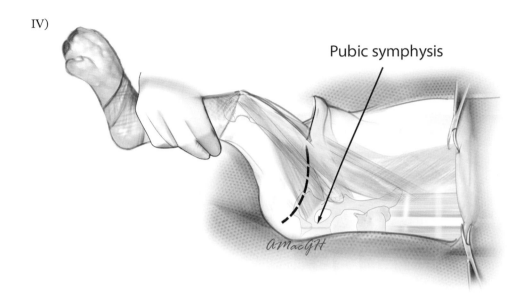

Pubic symphysis

V)

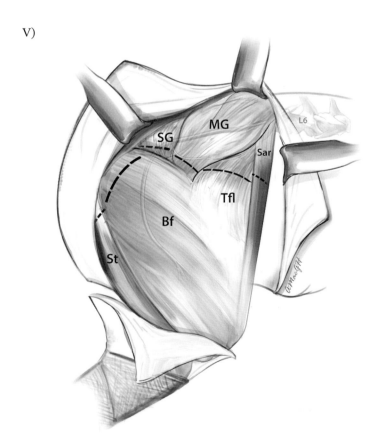

PATIENT POSITIONING AND DESCRIPTION OF THE PROCEDURE *continued*

VI) *Lateral dissection*

    Cranial: the osteotomy of the ilium is caudal to the sacroiliac joint, approximately at the level of the greater ischiatic notch. The iliopsoas and sartorius are elevated off the ilium ventrally and the medial gluteal muscle is partly elevated off the ilial wing at the planned site for the osteotomy and transected in order to expose the bone for an osteotomy.

    Caudal: the osteotomy of the ischium is caudal to the acetabulum, approximately at the level of the lesser ischiatic notch.

    The following structures are shown for orientation: adductor (Ad), gemelli (gem.), gracilis (Gr), biceps femoris (Bf), middle gluteal (MG), tensor fascia lata (Tfl), sartorius (Sar), and quadratus femoris (Qf) muscles and the sciatic nerve.

VII) After the osteotomies are completed, any remaining muscle and fascial attachments are dissected away and the pelvic bone and hind leg are removed en bloc.

CLOSURE

This is started by suturing the iliac muscles (iliopsoas, sartorius, and medial gluteal) over the defect and, if needed, reconstructing the abdominal wall and attaching the abdominal wall muscles either directly to the bone (using bone tunnels) or by using a mesh if needed. The remainder of the closure is performed by approximating the deeper layers first, followed by routine closure.

ALTERNATE POSITIONING AND APPROACHES

- A non-absorbable mesh might be needed to reconstruct the abdominal wall.
- The sartorius muscle can be used to close the defect.[20]
- The locations of the cranial and caudal cuts vary depending on the extent of the lesion and can be adjusted to include the entire ilial wing (cranial hemipelvectomy) or ipsilateral part of the ischium (caudal hemipelvectomy) if needed. A total (a), middle (acetabulectomy, b), and caudal hemipelvectomy (c) are shown highlighted.

Partial/Middle Hemipelvectomy (Acetabulectomy) *continued*

VI)

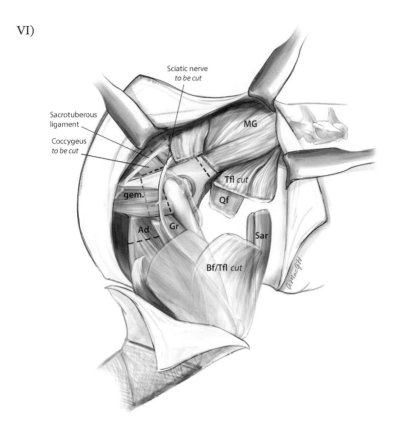

VII)

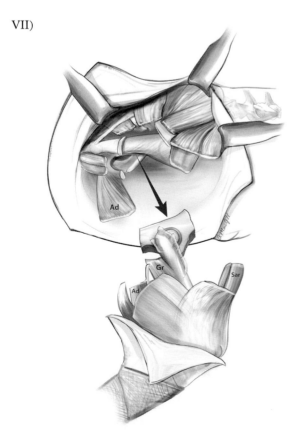

Total Hemipelvectomy[20-22]

INDICATIONS

- Total hemipelvectomy
- Total hemipelvectomy is illustrated in (a), whereas (b) and (c) depict a middle and caudal hemipelvectomy, respectively.

PATIENT POSITIONING AND DESCRIPTION OF THE PROCEDURE

I) The affected hindlimb, caudal abdomen, and lumbar area (extending to the contralateral side of midline) are clipped and prepped. The patient is placed in lateral recumbency with the affected leg uppermost in a hanging limb drape. The entire dorsal portion of the pelvis and caudal abdomen are draped in, allowing access circumferentially around the pelvis.

   The following structures are shown for orientation: semitendinosus (St), biceps femoris (BF), middle gluteal (MG), tensor fascia lata (TFL), sartorius (Sar), and epaxial (Epax) muscles and the sciatic (Sc) nerve. The ischium and ilium are similarly indicated.

Atlas of Surgical Approaches to Soft Tissue and Oncologic Diseases in the Dog and Cat, First Edition. Marije Risselada.
© 2020 John Wiley & Sons, Inc. Published 2020 by John Wiley & Sons, Inc.

Total Hemipelvectomy

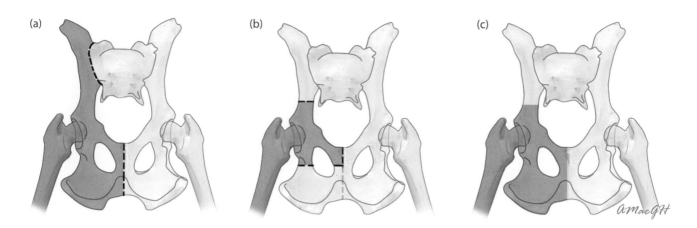

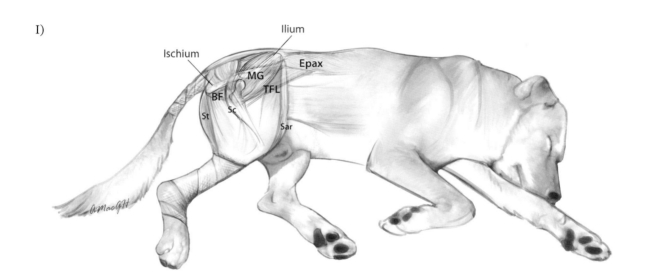

PATIENT POSITIONING AND DESCRIPTION OF THE PROCEDURE *continued*

II, III) The incision line is planned along the dorsolateral aspect of the hip and along the inguinal canal, ensuring enough skin dorsolaterally to close the defect without tension.

Total Hemipelvectomy *continued*

II)

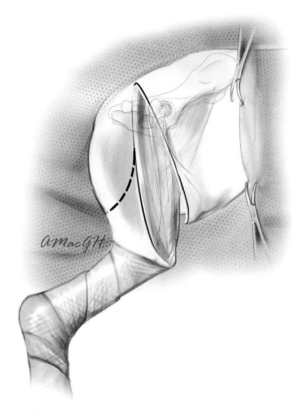

III)

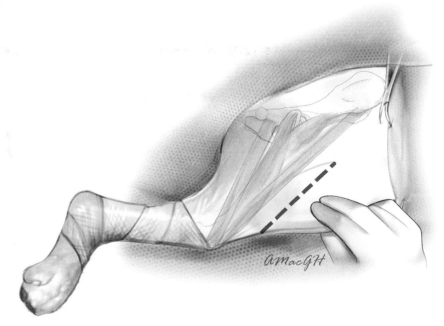

PATIENT POSITIONING AND DESCRIPTION OF THE PROCEDURE *continued*

IV) *Ventral dissection*: the subcutaneous tissues are dissected away from the midline to expose the medial thigh muscles (adductor, gracilis, and pectineus muscles). These muscles are transected and/or elevated off the bone to expose the midline of the pubis with sufficient exposure for an osteotomy. The insertions of the abdominal muscles are similarly elevated off the bone. After the osteotomy, the intrapelvic muscles are carefully elevated off the bone medially.

V) *Dorsal/dorsolateral dissection*

    Cranial: the skin is elevated to expose the biceps femoris (Bf), gluteal, and sartorial (Sar) muscles. The biceps femoris muscle is transected proximally. The sartorial muscle is transected to allow access to the medial side of the ilium and sacroiliac joint. This can be performed close to the ilium or further away (mid-body).

    The superficial gluteal (SG) muscle is isolated and transected close to its origin and reflected distally. The middle gluteal (MG) muscle is similarly elevated, but, if possible, it is transected closer to its insertion on the femur to save more muscle bulk for closure.

    The following other structures are shown for orientation: semitendinosus (St) and tensor fascia lata (Tfl).

Total Hemipelvectomy *continued*

IV)

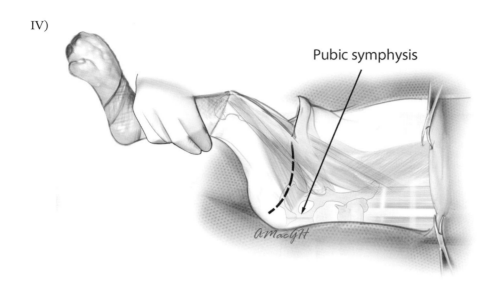

Pubic symphysis

V)

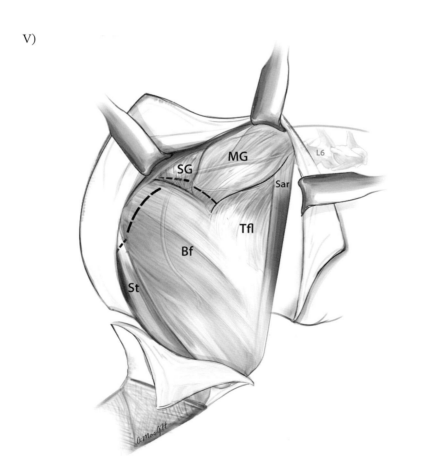

PATIENT POSITIONING AND DESCRIPTION OF THE PROCEDURE *continued*

VI) *Lateral dissection*

   Cranial: the deep gluteal muscle and piriform muscles are similarly transected. The craniodorsal aspect of the ilial wing is exposed by elevating muscles off the ilium. The sacroiliac joint is exposed by transecting the rectus femoris muscle near its origin. Ventrally the iliopsoas muscle is elevated at its insertion, after which the joint can be disarticulated.

   Caudal: caudally, the dissection is continued close to the ischium. The sacrotuberous ligament is transected and care is taken not to disrupt the levator ani and coccygeus muscles.

   The following structures are shown for orientation: adductor (Ad), gemelli (Gm), semitendinosus (St), biceps femoris (Bf), middle gluteal (MG), sartorius (Sar), gracilis (Gr), and quadratus femoris (Qtf) muscles.

VII) After the osteotomies are completed, any remaining muscle and fascial attachments are dissected away and the pelvic bone and hind leg are removed en bloc.

CLOSURE

The abdominal wall (Abdom) is reconstructed first by attaching the abdominal wall muscles either to any remaining muscles locally, directly to the bone of the symphysis (using bone tunnels), or by using a mesh if needed. The remainder of the closure is performed by approximating the deeper layers first, followed by routine closure.

ALTERNATE POSITIONING AND APPROACHES

- A non-absorbable mesh might be needed to reconstruct the abdominal wall.
- The sartorius muscle can be used to close the defect if its ilial attachment can be left intact.[20]
- The extent of the cranial part of the hemipelvectomy (total or subtotal) varies depending on the cranial extent of the lesion.
- If a piece of ilium can be left cranially, holes can be drilled to anchor sutures for reconstruction of the defect.

Total Hemipelvectomy *continued*

VI)

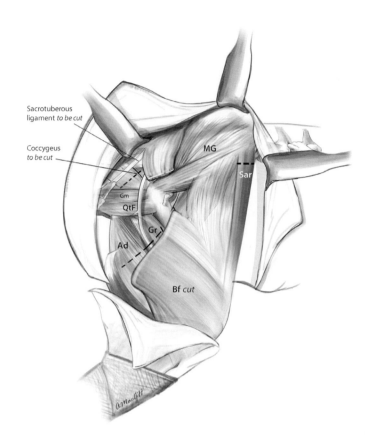

VII)

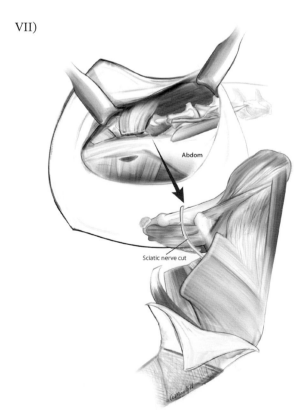

Coxofemoral Disarticulation[3,8,10]

INDICATIONS

- Trauma or neoplasia of the distal hindlimb

PATIENT POSITIONING AND DESCRIPTION OF THE PROCEDURE

I)   The affected hindlimb, caudal abdomen, and lumbar area (extending to the contralateral side of midline) are clipped and prepped. The patient is placed in lateral recumbency with the affected leg uppermost in a hanging limb drape, allowing full access to the limb during the procedure. A skin incision is planned at the coxofemoral joint with slightly more skin preserved laterally than inguinally, allowing for more tissue coverage from the lateral side than the medial side.

The following structures are shown for orientation: semitendinosus (St), biceps femoris (BF), middle gluteal (MG), tensor fascia lata (TFL), sartorius (Sar), and epaxial (Epax) muscles and the sciatic (Sc) nerve. The ischium and ilium are similarly indicated.

II) *Superficial dissection*

Medial: the subcutaneous tissues are dissected away to expose the Sartorius (Sar), pectineus, gracilis, and adductor muscles, which are transected. The femoral nerve is identified and transected after an intraneural block. The femoral artery and vein are identified, ligated, and transected.

Lateral: the subcutaneous tissues are dissected away to expose the biceps femoris (Bf), abductor, and tensor fascia lata muscles (Tfl). The muscles are transected away from their origins (i.e. as close to the hip/femur as possible) to allow for muscles to remain attached for closure.

The superficial (SG), middle gluteal (MG), and semitendinosus (St) muscles are depicted for orientation.

Atlas of Surgical Approaches to Soft Tissue and Oncologic Diseases in the Dog and Cat, First Edition. Marije Risselada.
© 2020 John Wiley & Sons, Inc. Published 2020 by John Wiley & Sons, Inc.

Coxofemoral Disarticulation

I)

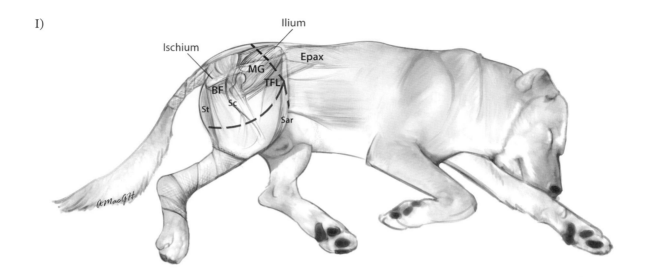

II)

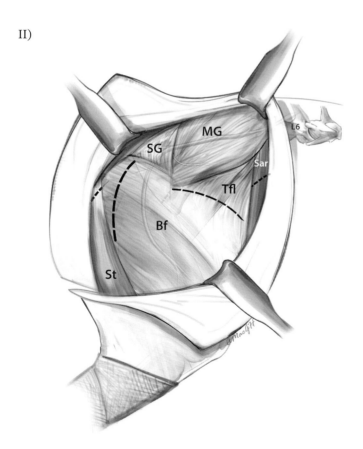

PATIENT POSITIONING AND DESCRIPTION OF THE PROCEDURE *continued*

III) *Deep dissection*: the muscles are reflected dorsally to expose the coxofemoral joint. The semitendinosus and semimembranosus muscles are transected, as is the sciatic nerve.

   The remaining muscles (quadratus femoris, external rotators, gluteal muscles) are cut near their femoral attachments.

   The following muscles are shown: adductor (Ad), gracilis (Gr), middle gluteal (MG), adductor (Ad), biceps femoris (Bf), tensor fascia lata (Tfl), gemelli (Gm), quadratus femoris (Qtf), and quadriceps femoris (QcF).

IV) The joint capsule is incised, the teres ligament transected, and the amputation completed.

CLOSURE

First the deeper tissues and muscles are approximated to reconstruct and cover the acetabulum, after which the subcutaneous tissues and skin are closed routinely.

ALTERNATE POSITIONING AND APPROACHES

- A mid-femoral amputation is an alternative for lesions below the stifle.
- For even more proximal lesions, an acetabulectomy or (total) hemipelvectomy can be considered.

Coxofemoral Disarticulation *continued*

III)

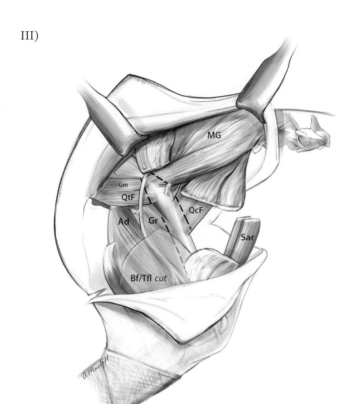

IV)

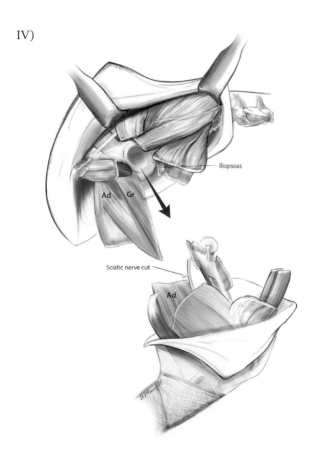

Mid-Femoral Amputation[1,3,10,17]

INDICATIONS

- Trauma or neoplasia of the distal hindlimb

PATIENT POSITIONING AND DESCRIPTION OF THE PROCEDURE

I,II) The affected hindlimb, caudal abdomen, and lumbar area (extending to the contralateral side of midline) are clipped and prepped. The patient is placed in lateral recumbency with the affected leg uppermost in a hanging limb drape, allowing full access to the limb during the procedure. A skin incision is planned at the level of the stifle, or just proximal to the stifle, allowing for more tissue coverage from the lateral side than the medial side.

The biceps femoris (BF) muscle is indicated for orientation.

Atlas of Surgical Approaches to Soft Tissue and Oncologic Diseases in the Dog and Cat, First Edition. Marije Risselada.
© 2020 John Wiley & Sons, Inc. Published 2020 by John Wiley & Sons, Inc.

Mid-Femoral Amputation

I)

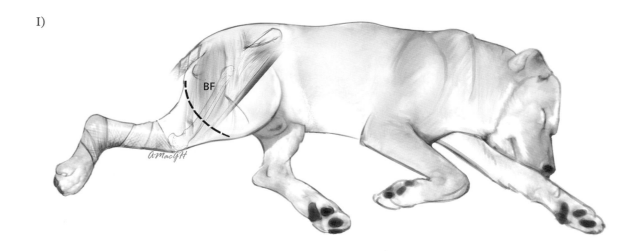

II)

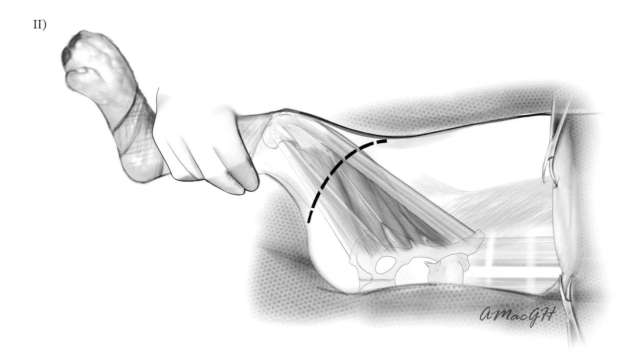

PATIENT POSITIONING AND DESCRIPTION OF THE PROCEDURE *continued*

III) The skin is incised and reflected dorsally, exposing the tensor fascia lata (Tfl), vastus lateralis and biceps femoris (Bf) muscles laterally as well as the sartorius (Sar) muscles cranially and semimembranosus and semitendinosus (St) muscle caudally. These muscles are transected near their insertions in order to preserve as much muscle belly as possible to protect the stump.

IV) The semitendinosus (St) and gracilis (Gr) muscles are similarly transected. Dissection is continued along the femur proximally, elevating the adductor (Ad) and vastus medialis muscles off their femoral insertions close to the bone. This is continued dorsally to the site of the planned osteotomy, at a level just distal to the lesser trochanter.

Mid-Femoral Amputation *continued*

III)

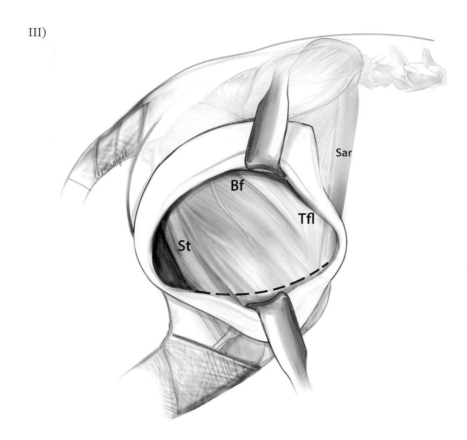

IV)

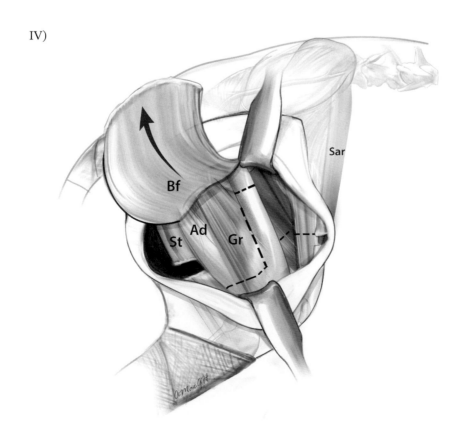

CLOSURE

V)   After ensuring the smoothness of the osteotomy line, closure is started by folding muscles over the stump and suturing the muscles in place, starting with the deeper muscles and gradually working towards the more peripheral muscles, such as the semitendinosus (St) and Sartorius (Sar). If a larger portion of the biceps femoris (Bf) is left, it can be used to fold over the stump as additional bulk. The remainder of the closure is routine.

ALTERNATE POSITIONING AND APPROACHES

- A coxofemoral disarticulation is an alternative if the neoplasia involves the stifle or femur. Transection of muscles further away from the stifle can be performed if more margin distally is desired.
- For even more proximal lesions, a hemipelvectomy can be considered.

Mid-Femoral Amputation *continued*

V)

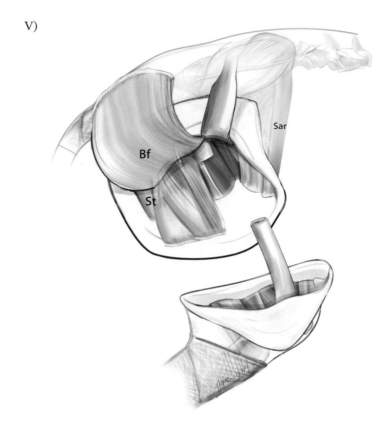

Approach to the Popliteal Lymph Node[3,17]

INDICATIONS

- Popliteal lymph node biopsy
- Popliteal lymph node removal

PATIENT POSITIONING AND DESCRIPTION OF THE PROCEDURE

I) The caudal area of the hind leg from ischium to mid-tibia is clipped and prepared, extending laterally and medially around the stifle area. The patient is placed in lateral recumbency with the affected leg uppermost. The leg can be positioned and draped in a hanging limb position, or only the popliteal area can be clipped, prepped, and draped. A skin incision is centered over the popliteal lymph node (LN), over the caudal aspect of the hindlimb.

   The semitendinosus muscle and saphenous (Saph) artery and vein are shown.

II) The subcutaneous tissues are bluntly dissected to expose the lymph node that lies in between the biceps femoris and semitendinosus muscles. For removal, the lymph node is retracted and dissected away from its tissue attachments and removed.

CLOSURE

The muscles and deeper tissues are apposed to close dead space. The remainder of the closure is routine.

ALTERNATE POSITIONING AND APPROACHES

- Placing a traction suture through the lymph node can facilitate in retraction and resection.
- The skin incision can be extended if needed to facilitate removal of an enlarged lymph node.

Atlas of Surgical Approaches to Soft Tissue and Oncologic Diseases in the Dog and Cat, First Edition. Marije Risselada.
© 2020 John Wiley & Sons, Inc. Published 2020 by John Wiley & Sons, Inc.

Approach to the Popliteal Lymph Node

I)

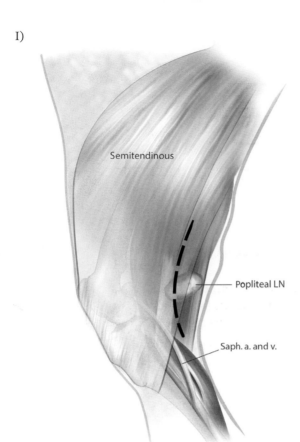

II)

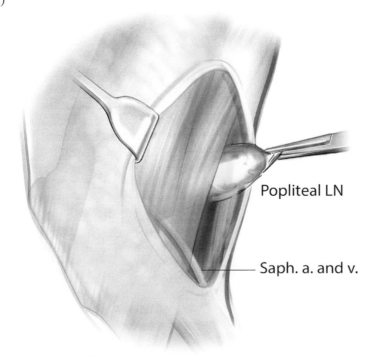

Approach to the Femoral Artery[3,17]

INDICATIONS

- Femoral artery access for interventional procedures
- Femoral artery ligation – temporary or permanent

PATIENT POSITIONING AND DESCRIPTION OF THE PROCEDURE

I) The medial thigh area, inguinal area, and ventral abdomen are clipped and prepared. The patient is placed in (dorso) lateral recumbency with the affected leg down and the other leg pulled forward or retracted dorsally. A skin incision is made along the long axis of the femur, in the triangular area in between the sartorius muscle (cranially), the pectineus muscle (caudally), and the pelvis (medially).

II) The sartorius muscle is retracted cranially to expose the femoral artery, vein, and nerve. The femoral artery is dissected away from the vein and the nerve.

CLOSURE

After the procedure the incision is closed routinely.

ALTERNATE POSITIONING AND APPROACHES

- This can be performed with the patient in dorsal recumbency with the appropriate hind leg draped in, if dorsal recumbency is needed for concurrent procedures, avoiding having to reposition the patient.

Atlas of Surgical Approaches to Soft Tissue and Oncologic Diseases in the Dog and Cat, First Edition. Marije Risselada.
© 2020 John Wiley & Sons, Inc. Published 2020 by John Wiley & Sons, Inc.

Approach to the Femoral Artery

I)

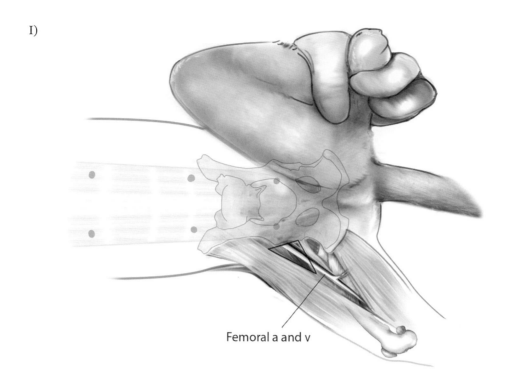

Femoral a and v

II)

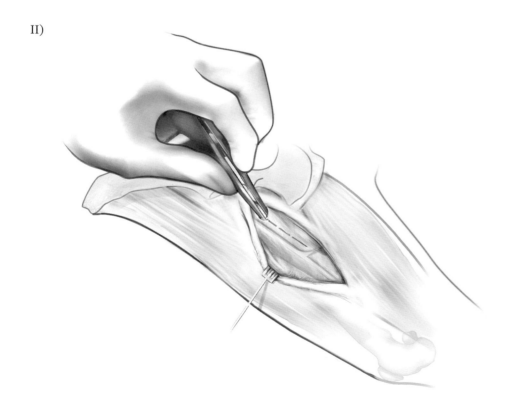

Section 5

Thorax

Right Lateral Approach to the Cranial Thorax[3,16]

INDICATIONS

- Access to the esophagus, right cranial lung lobe
- Access to heart and pericardium
- Access to the cranial mediastinum

PATIENT POSITIONING AND DESCRIPTION OF THE PROCEDURE

I) The patient is placed in left lateral recumbency with the right leg pulled forward. The lateral thorax is clipped and prepared from the axillary region to caudal to the last rib, extending dorsal to the spinous processes and ventral to the sternum. The incision is centered over the 5th intercostal space.

II) The subcutaneous tissues are bluntly dissected and the cutaneous trunci muscle is transected to expose the latissimus dorsi muscle covering the dorsal part of the incision. The fascial attachments along the ventral attachment of the latissimus dorsi muscle are transected, allowing dorsal retraction of the muscle.[a] If additional (dorsal) exposure is needed, the ventral portion of the muscle can be transected along the line of the incision and ribs.

---

[a]Transection of the latissimus dorsi is shown in the Left Lateral Approach to the Cranial Thorax.

Atlas of Surgical Approaches to Soft Tissue and Oncologic Diseases in the Dog and Cat, First Edition. Marije Risselada.
© 2020 John Wiley & Sons, Inc. Published 2020 by John Wiley & Sons, Inc.

Right Lateral Approach to the Cranial Thorax

I)

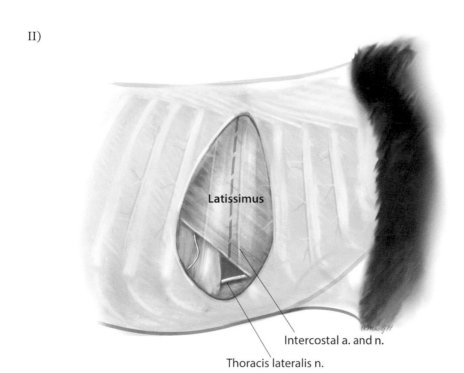

II)

PATIENT POSITIONING AND DESCRIPTION OF THE PROCEDURE *continued*

III) The individual muscle bellies of the serratus ventralis are divided to obtain access to the intercostal space. The scalenus muscle inserts on the cranial aspect of the 6th rib and will need to be transected. The external and internal intercostal muscles are elevated with a forceps and are transected (dashed line) in the middle of the intercostal space, taking care to avoid the intercostal artery (ia) and nerve (ic) at the caudal aspect of the ribs.

Retraction of the ribs allows access to the intrathoracic structures, such as the pericardium, the cranial lung lobes, and the cranial esophagus, after ventral retraction of the cranial vena cava.

The abdominal oblique (Abd obl), scalenus (Scal), and serratus muscles are shown for orientation.

CLOSURE

A thoracostomy tube is placed prior to closure. Encircling sutures are preplaced around the ribs cranial and caudal to the incision and tightened to appose the ribs. The intercostal muscles can be closed in a separate simple continuous fashion, after which the remainder of the incision is closed routinely.

ALTERNATE POSITIONING AND APPROACHES

- The planned intercostal space for the thoracotomy can be changed based on the exact location of the intrathoracic structures of interest.

Right Lateral Approach to the Cranial Thorax *continued*

III)

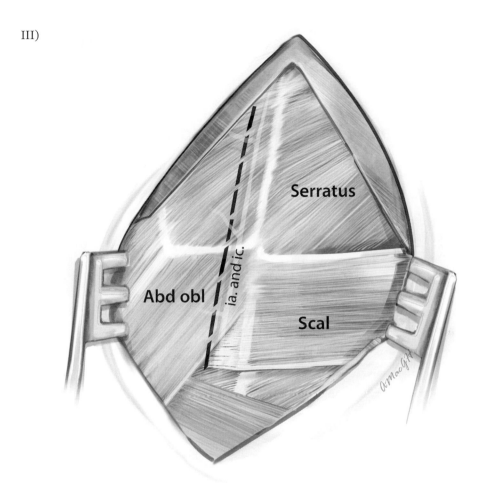

Left Lateral Approach to the Cranial Thorax[3,16]

INDICATIONS

- Access to cranial lung lobe, thymus, heart
- Access to heart and pericardial procedures for:
  - Ligation of a patent ductus arteriosum
  - Division of a persistent right aortic arch
  - Epicardial pacemaker placement

PATIENT POSITIONING AND DESCRIPTION OF THE PROCEDURE

I) The patient is placed in left lateral recumbency with the right leg pulled forward. The lateral thorax is clipped and prepared from the axillary region to caudal to the last rib, extending dorsal to the spinous processes and ventral to the sternum. The incision is centered over the 4th intercostal space.

II) The subcutaneous tissues are bluntly dissected and the cutaneous trunci muscle is transected to expose the latissimus dorsi muscle (Lat) covering the dorsal part of the incision. The fascial attachments along the ventral attachment of the latissimus dorsi muscle are transected, allowing dorsal retraction of the muscle. If additional (dorsal) exposure is needed, the ventral portion of the muscle can be transected along the line of the incision and ribs.[a]

---

[a] Transection of the latissimus dorsi is shown in Right Lateral Approach to the Cranial Thorax.

Atlas of Surgical Approaches to Soft Tissue and Oncologic Diseases in the Dog and Cat, First Edition. Marije Risselada.
© 2020 John Wiley & Sons, Inc. Published 2020 by John Wiley & Sons, Inc.

Left Lateral Approach to the Cranial Thorax

I)

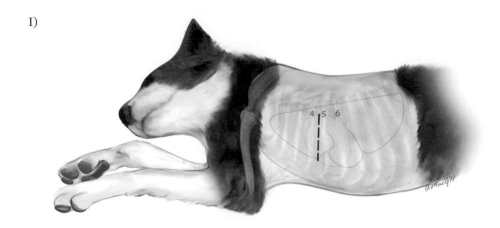

II)

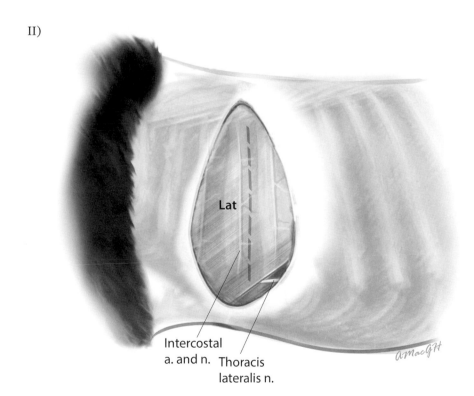

Lat

Intercostal
a. and n.   Thoracis
lateralis n.

PATIENT POSITIONING AND DESCRIPTION OF THE PROCEDURE *continued*

III) The individual muscle bellies of the serratus ventralis muscle (Ser) are divided to obtain access to the intercostal space. The scalenus muscle (Scal) inserts on the cranial aspect of the 6th rib and will need to be transected. The external and internal intercostal muscles are elevated with a forceps and are transected in the middle of the intercostal space, taking care to avoid the intercostal artery (ia) and nerve (ic) at the caudal aspect of the ribs.

Retraction of the ribs allows access to the intrathoracic structures, including the thymus and ligamentum/ductus arteriosum.

CLOSURE

A thoracostomy tube is placed prior to closure. Encircling sutures are preplaced around the ribs cranial and caudal to the incision and tightened to appose the ribs. The intercostal muscles can be closed in a separate simple continuous fashion, after which the remainder of the incision is closed routinely.

ALTERNATE POSITIONING AND APPROACHES

- The planned intercostal space for the thoracotomy can be changed based on the exact location of the intrathoracic structures of interest.

Left Lateral Approach to the Cranial Thorax *continued*

III)

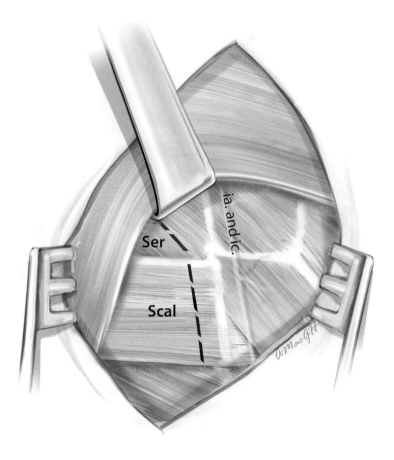

Right Lateral Approach to the Caudal Thorax[3,16]

INDICATIONS

- Access to caudal lung lobes
- Thoracic duct ligation in the dog
- Esophagotomy

PATIENT POSITIONING AND DESCRIPTION OF THE PROCEDURE

I) The patient is placed in left lateral recumbency with the right leg pulled forward. The lateral thorax is clipped and prepared from the axillary region to caudal to the last rib, extending dorsal to the spinous processes and ventral to the sternum. The incision is centered over the 9th intercostal space.

II) The subcutaneous tissues are bluntly dissected and the cutaneous trunci muscle is transected to expose the latissimus dorsi muscle (Lat) covering the dorsal part of the incision. The fascial attachments along the ventral attachment of the latissimus dorsi muscle are transected, allowing dorsal retraction of the muscle. If additional (dorsal) exposure is needed, the ventral portion of the muscle can be transected along the line of the incision and ribs. The external and internal intercostal muscles are elevated with a forceps and are transected in the middle of the intercostal space, taking care to avoid the intercostal artery and nerve at the caudal aspect of the ribs.

Atlas of Surgical Approaches to Soft Tissue and Oncologic Diseases in the Dog and Cat, First Edition. Marije Risselada.
© 2020 John Wiley & Sons, Inc. Published 2020 by John Wiley & Sons, Inc.

Right Lateral Approach to the Caudal Thorax

I)

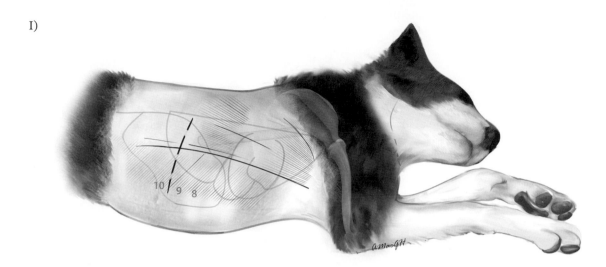

II)

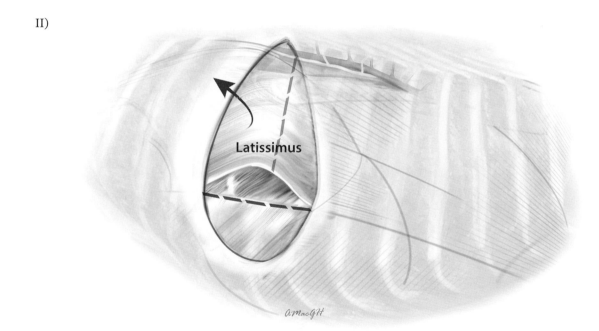

PATIENT POSITIONING AND DESCRIPTION OF THE PROCEDURE *continued*

III) Retraction of the ribs allows access to the intrathoracic structures, including the thoracic duct and diaphragm (Dp). Ribs 9 (r9) and 10 (r10) are indicated.

CLOSURE

A thoracostomy tube is placed prior to closure. Encircling sutures are preplaced around the ribs cranial and caudal to the incision and tightened to appose the ribs. The intercostal muscles can be closed in a separate simple continuous fashion, after which the remainder of the incision is closed routinely.

ALTERNATE POSITIONING AND APPROACHES

- The planned intercostal space for the thoracotomy can be changed based on the exact location of the intrathoracic structures of interest.
- The pericardium and heart can be reached from a caudal thoracotomy approach, but a second, more cranial thoracotomy might be preferred to obtain better access.
- An esophagotomy can be performed via left or right caudal thoracotomy.

Right Lateral Approach to the Caudal Thorax *continued*

III)

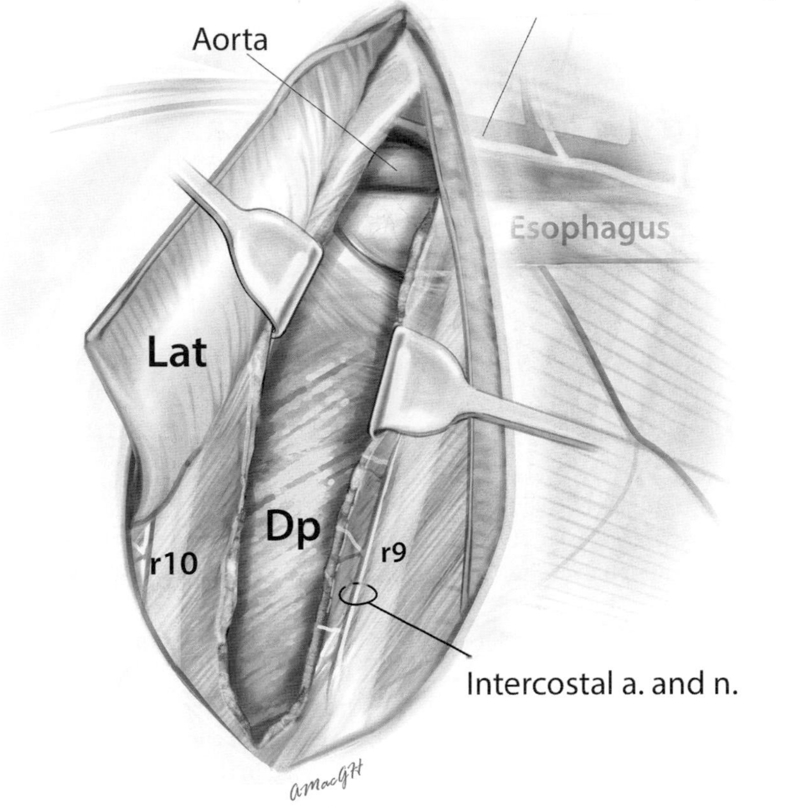

Thoracic duct passes behind diaphragm

Aorta

Esophagus

Lat

Dp

r10

r9

Intercostal a. and n.

Left Lateral Approach to the Caudal Thorax[3,16]

INDICATIONS

- Access to the caudal lung lobes
- Esophagotomy

PATIENT POSITIONING AND DESCRIPTION OF THE PROCEDURE

I)   The patient is placed in right lateral recumbency with the left leg pulled forward. The lateral thorax is clipped and prepared from the axillary region to caudal to the last rib, extending dorsal to the spinous processes and ventral to the sternum. The incision is centered over the 9th intercostal space. Ribs 9 and 10 are indicated, as is the caudal vena cava (CVC).

II) The subcutaneous tissues are bluntly dissected and the cutaneous trunci muscle is transected to expose the latissimus dorsi muscle covering the dorsal part of the incision. The fascial attachments along the ventral attachment of the latissimus dorsi muscle are transected, allowing dorsal retraction of the muscle. If additional (dorsal) exposure is needed, the ventral portion of the muscle can be transected along the line of the incision and ribs. The external and internal intercostal muscles are elevated with a forceps and are transected in the middle of the intercostal space, taking care to avoid the intercostal artery and nerve at the caudal aspect of the ribs. The diaphragm is indicated with Dp.

III) Retraction of the ribs allows access to the intrathoracic structures, including the esophagus and caudal vena cava.

CLOSURE

A thoracostomy tube is placed prior to closure. Encircling sutures are preplaced around the ribs cranial and caudal to the incision and tightened to appose the ribs. The intercostal muscles can be closed in a separate simple continuous fashion, after which the remainder of the incision is closed routinely.

ALTERNATE POSITIONING AND APPROACHES

- The planned intercostal space for the thoracotomy can be changed based on the exact location of the intrathoracic structures of interest. The pericardium and heart can be reached from a caudal thoracotomy approach, but a second, more cranial thoracotomy might be preferred to obtain better access.
- Epicardial pacemaker placement can be performed via a caudal or more cranial left lateral thoracotomy or via a transdiaphragmatic approach.
- An esophagotomy can be performed via left or right caudal thoracotomy.

Atlas of Surgical Approaches to Soft Tissue and Oncologic Diseases in the Dog and Cat, First Edition. Marije Risselada.
© 2020 John Wiley & Sons, Inc. Published 2020 by John Wiley & Sons, Inc.

Left Lateral Approach to the Caudal Thorax

I)

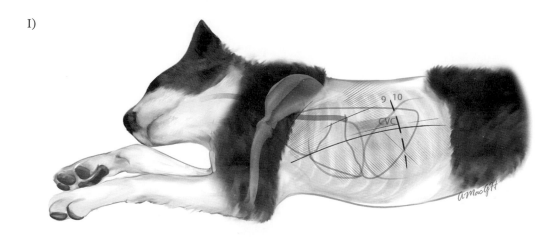

II)

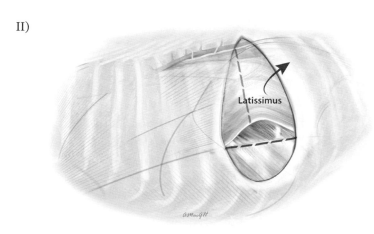

III)

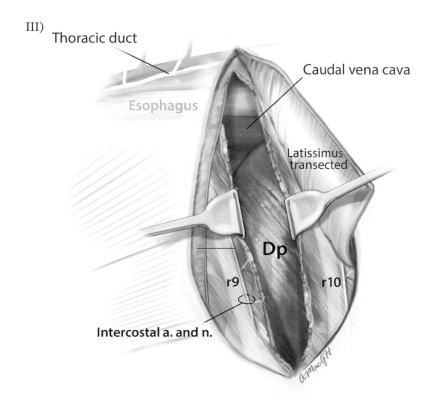

Closure of a Rib Wall Resection without Diaphragmatic Advancement[3,16]

INDICATIONS

- Thoracic wall neoplasia

PATIENT POSITIONING AND DESCRIPTION OF THE PROCEDURE

I) The patient is placed in lateral recumbency with the font leg pulled forward. The lateral thorax is clipped and prepared from the axillary region to caudal to the last rib, extending dorsal to the spinous processes and ventral to the sternum. The incision is centered around the planned resection site.

     The ribs and diaphragm (Dp) below are schematically indicated in the defect site.

II) The subcutaneous tissues are bluntly dissected and the cutaneous trunci muscle is transected or resected (depending on the margin requirement of the mass) to expose the latissimus dorsi muscle covering the dorsal part of the incision. The latissimus dorsi muscle is either transected or resected (for tumor margins, similar to the more superficial incision). The external and internal intercostal muscles of the proposed intercostal spaces cranial and caudal to the mass are elevated with a forceps and are transected in the middle of the intercostal space, taking care to avoid the intercostal artery and nerve at the caudal aspect of the ribs. A similar window is made for each intercostal space along the dorsal and ventral margin of the proposed resection site. Intercostal nerve blocks are placed for each rib to be transected. The ribs are transected dorsally and ventrally, and the segment is lifted away from the thorax.

Atlas of Surgical Approaches to Soft Tissue and Oncologic Diseases in the Dog and Cat, First Edition. Marije Risselada.
© 2020 John Wiley & Sons, Inc. Published 2020 by John Wiley & Sons, Inc.

Closure of a Rib Wall Resection without Diaphragmatic Advancement

I)

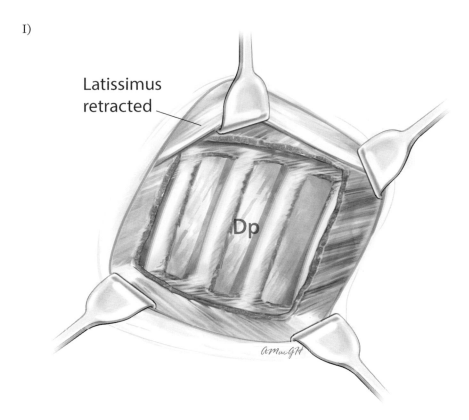

II)

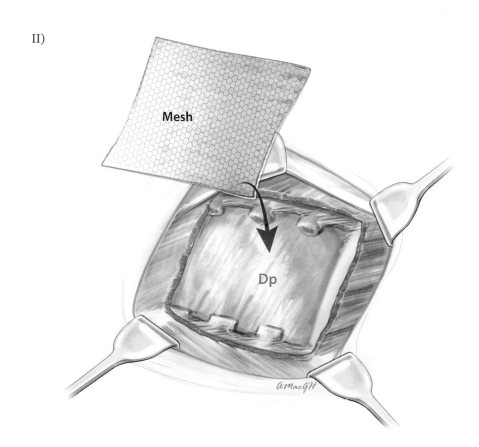

CLOSURE

III) Mesh is placed in the defect and sutured to the soft tissue structures surrounding the defect. Circumcostal sutures cranially and caudally will aid in the security of the mesh placement. The edges of the mesh can either be laid flat or doubled over to avoid rubbing on and traumatizing the subcutaneous tissues and skin. The remaining muscles are used to try to cover the mesh as much as possible. The subcutaneous tissues and skin are closed routinely.

ALTERNATE POSITIONING AND APPROACHES

- The planned intercostal space for the thoracotomy can be changed based on the exact location of the intrathoracic structures of interest.
- For a caudal rib resection, a diaphragmatic advancement could be utilized.

Closure of a Rib Wall Resection without Diaphragmatic Advancement *continued*

III)

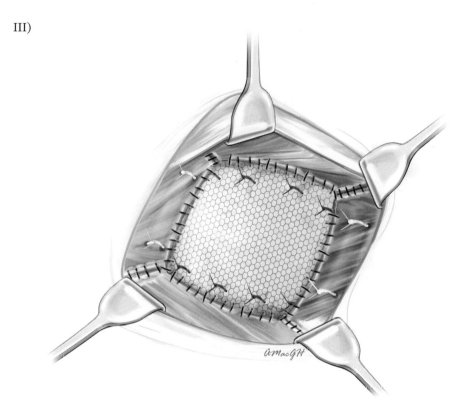

Closure of a Rib Wall Resection with Diaphragmatic Advancement[3,16,23]

INDICATIONS

- Chest wall with/without diaphragmatic mass resections

PATIENT POSITIONING AND DESCRIPTION OF THE PROCEDURE

I) The patient is placed in lateral recumbency with the font leg pulled forward. The lateral thorax and cranial portion of the lateral abdomen are clipped and prepared from the axillary region to caudal to the last rib, extending dorsal to the spinous processes and ventral to the sternum. The incision is centered around the planned resection site.

   The diaphragm (Dp) is shown from the abdominal side.

II) The subcutaneous tissues are bluntly dissected and the cutaneous trunci muscle is transected or resected (depending on the margin requirement of the mass) to expose the latissimus dorsi muscle covering the dorsal part of the incision. The latissimus dorsi muscle is either transected or resected (for tumor margins, similar to the more superficial incision). The external and internal intercostal muscles of the proposed intercostal spaces cranial and caudal to the mass are elevated with a forceps and are transected in the middle of the intercostal space, taking care to avoid the intercostal artery and nerve at the caudal aspect of the ribs. A similar window is made for each intercostal space along the dorsal and ventral margin of the proposed resection site. Intercostal nerve blocks are placed for each rib to be transected. The ribs are transected dorsally and ventrally and the segment is lifted away from the thorax.

Atlas of Surgical Approaches to Soft Tissue and Oncologic Diseases in the Dog and Cat, First Edition. Marije Risselada.
© 2020 John Wiley & Sons, Inc. Published 2020 by John Wiley & Sons, Inc.

Closure of a Rib Wall Resection with Diaphragmatic Advancement

I)

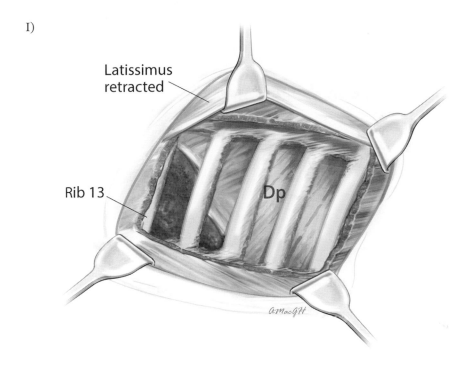

II)

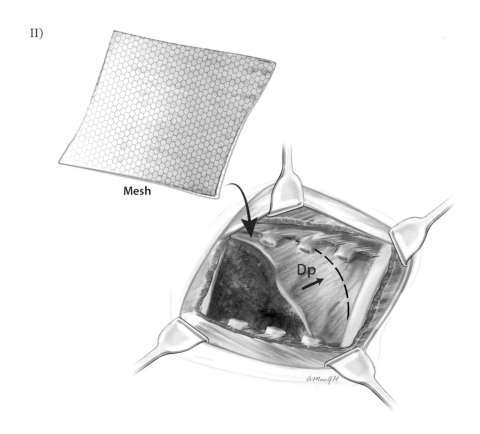

CLOSURE

III) The diaphragm is dissected away from its lateral attachments and advanced cranially by anchoring it to a rib (using circumcostal sutures) and musculature. A thoracostomy tube is placed prior to advancing the diaphragm.

    The body wall is reconstructed using muscle or mesh, after which the soft tissues are closed routinely.

ALTERNATE POSITIONING AND APPROACHES

- The caudal lung lobe might need to be removed to allow advancement of the diaphragm and closure.
- If needed, mesh can be used to reconstruct the body wall.

Closure of a Rib Wall Resection with Diaphragmatic Advancement *continued*

III)

Median Sternotomy[16]

INDICATIONS

- Thoracic exploratory surgery
- Thymectomy
- (Sub)total pericardiectomy

PATIENT POSITIONING AND DESCRIPTION OF THE PROCEDURE

I) The patient is placed in dorsal recumbency with the legs pulled forward. The ventral cervical, thoracic, and abdominal areas are clipped and prepped. The prepared area should extend more dorsally to accommodate thoracostomy tube placement, if desired. The incision is planned in midline, over the length of the sternum.

II,III) The subcutaneous tissues are bluntly dissected to expose the superficial and deep pectoral muscles. The sternebrae are exposed by elevating the muscles off the midline using a periosteal elevator, allowing better purchase for the osteotomy.

Atlas of Surgical Approaches to Soft Tissue and Oncologic Diseases in the Dog and Cat, First Edition. Marije Risselada.
© 2020 John Wiley & Sons, Inc. Published 2020 by John Wiley & Sons, Inc.

Median Sternotomy

I)

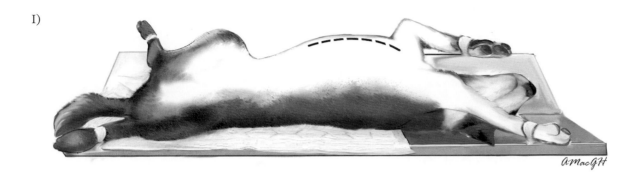

II)

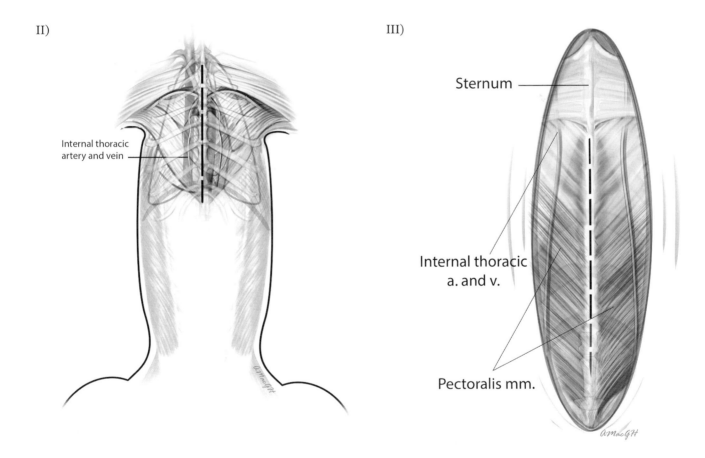

Internal thoracic
artery and vein

III)

Sternum

Internal thoracic
a. and v.

Pectoralis mm.

PATIENT POSITIONING AND DESCRIPTION OF THE PROCEDURE *continued*

IV) The osteotomy can be performed with an oscillating saw or osteotome and mallet, taking care to stay on midline, in order to avoid the internal thoracic arteries that run alongside the sternebrae.

CLOSURE

This is performed by reapposing the cut sternebrae using cerclage wire or heavy gauge suture (in smaller patients).

ALTERNATE POSITIONING AND APPROACHES

- The xiphoid and manubrium can be left intact for thoracic exploratory surgery in order to increase stability postoperatively. The incision can be centered cranially for increased exposure to the thoracic inlet, leaving the last sternebra and xiphoid intact. The incision can be centered caudally (combined with an abdominal midline incision), leaving the manubrium and first sternebra intact.
- An alternative approach to perform a subtotal pericardiectomy is from a right-sided intercostal thoracotomy.

Median Sternotomy *continued*

IV)

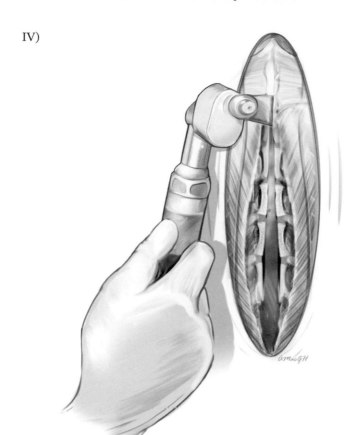

Transdiaphragmatic Approach to the Thorax[3,24]

INDICATIONS

- Epicardial pacemaker

PATIENT POSITIONING AND DESCRIPTION OF THE PROCEDURE

I) The patient is placed in dorsal recumbency with the caudoventral thorax and ventral abdomen clipped, prepped, and draped. The skin incision is planned along the cranial midline of the abdomen.

II) The subcutaneous tissues are dissected away from the fascia of the external abdominal oblique muscles on each side of the linea alba. A stab incision is made into the linea alba, while elevating the linea. The incision is lengthened cranially with either scissors or using a blade and groove director.

Atlas of Surgical Approaches to Soft Tissue and Oncologic Diseases in the Dog and Cat, First Edition. Marije Risselada.
© 2020 John Wiley & Sons, Inc. Published 2020 by John Wiley & Sons, Inc.

Transdiaphragmatic Approach to the Thorax

I)

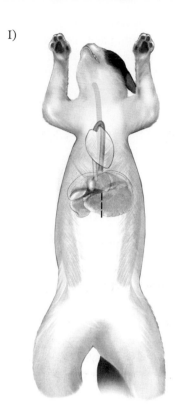

II)

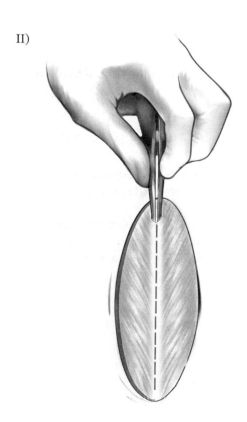

PATIENT POSITIONING AND DESCRIPTION OF THE PROCEDURE *continued*

III) Cranially the falciform ligament is identified and is resected. The liver (Lv) is protected by moistened laparotomy sponges and gently retracted dorsally and caudally using malleable retractors. The diaphragm (Dp) is grasped and a small incision is made in the muscular portion between the sternum and tendinous portion. This incision is lengthened in a dorsoventral direction using scissors. Stay sutures are placed on either side to retract the edges and facilitate exposure of intrathoracic structures.

CLOSURE

IV) This starts by approximating both sides of the diaphragmatic incision similar to a diaphragmatic hernia repair. A thoracostomy tube can be placed prior to closure, or alternatively can be placed in the diaphragmatic incision and removed after establishing negative intrathoracic pressure. The remainder of the abdominal closure is routine.

Transdiaphragmatic Approach to the Thorax *continued*

III)

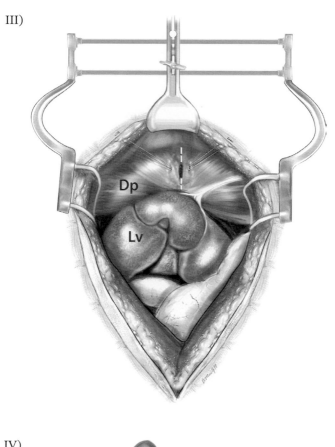

IV)

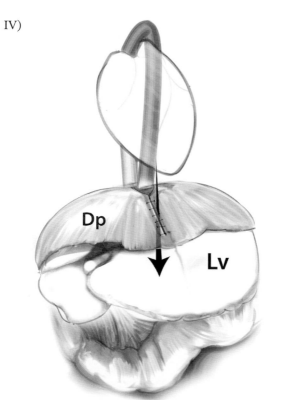

ALTERNATE POSITIONING AND APPROACHES

- If needed, more access can be obtained by adding a caudal median sternotomy.

V) In cases with diaphragmatic hernia, the defect in the diaphragm might need to be enlarged to allow reduction of the intraabdominal organs from the chest into the abdomen.

Transdiaphragmatic Approach to the Thorax *continued*

V)

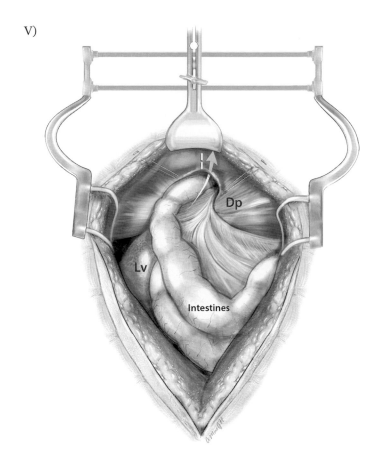

Section 6

Abdomen

Midline Approach to the Abdomen (Female Dog, Cats)[3,17]

INDICATIONS

- Abdominal exploratory surgery

PATIENT POSITIONING AND DESCRIPTION OF THE PROCEDURE

I, II) The patient is placed in dorsal recumbency with the ventral abdomen clipped and prepped from cranial to the xiphoid to caudal to the pubis, extending dorsally to mid-abdomen on the left and right side. The ventral midline is draped, leaving an area open extending cranially and caudally to the intended skin incision. The skin incision is planned along the midline.

Atlas of Surgical Approaches to Soft Tissue and Oncologic Diseases in the Dog and Cat, First Edition. Marije Risselada.
© 2020 John Wiley & Sons, Inc. Published 2020 by John Wiley & Sons, Inc.

Midline Approach to the Abdomen (Female Dog, Cats)

I)

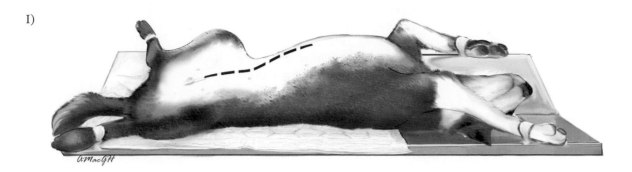

II)

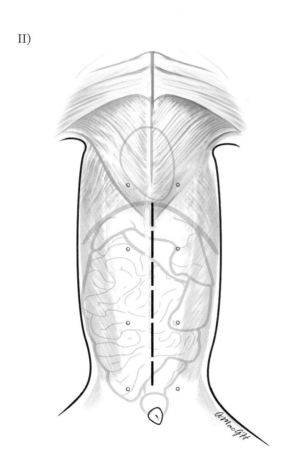

PATIENT POSITIONING AND DESCRIPTION OF THE PROCEDURE *continued*

III) The subcutaneous tissues are dissected away from the fascia of the external abdominal oblique muscles on each side of the linea alba. A stab incision is made into the linea alba, while elevating the linea. The incision is lengthened cranially and caudally either with scissors or using a blade and groove director.

IV) Cranially the falciform ligament is seen. This can be either removed or reflected to the non-surgeon side.
    The image shows the liver (LV), stomach and intestines for illustrative purposes.

CLOSURE

Both sides of the incision are approximated, taking deep bites of the fascia and the linea and avoiding full thickness bites or incorporation of the peritoneal layer. The remainder of the closure is routine. This involves a subcutaneous layer, skin closure, with/without a deeper layer as needed based on body conformation/condition. The subcutaneous layer(s) can incorporate bites to the fascial layer, eliminating/minimizing dead space if desired.

ALTERNATE POSITIONING AND APPROACHES

- The skin incision can extend from the xiphoid to the pubis or can center only on the cranial, middle, or caudal abdomen.
- If needed, more access can be obtained by adding a caudal median sternotomy or a paracostal approach.

Midline Approach to the Abdomen (Female Dog, Cats) *continued*

III)

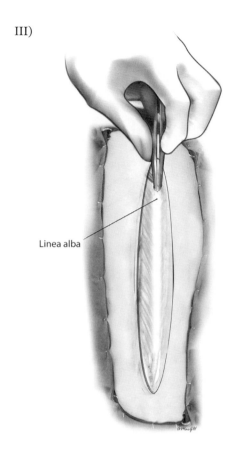

Linea alba

IV)

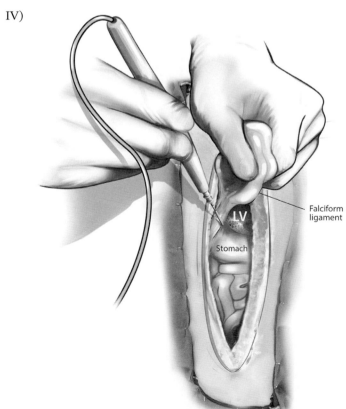

Falciform
ligament

LV

Stomach

Midline Approach to the Abdomen (Male Dog)[3,17]

INDICATIONS

- Abdominal exploratory surgery in male dogs

PATIENT POSITIONING AND DESCRIPTION OF THE PROCEDURE

I) The patient is placed in dorsal recumbency with the ventral abdomen clipped and prepped from cranial to the xiphoid to caudal to the pubis, extending dorsally to mid-abdomen on the left and right side. The prepuce can be draped in if access is needed for urinary surgery or can be reflected and draped out of the incision. The skin incision is planned along the midline, curving around the prepuce towards the surgeon (right side of the dog for a right-handed surgeon) and leaving enough space between the preputial orifice and the incision to allow for tension-free closure and to minimize urine scalding.

II, III) The subcutaneous tissues are dissected away from the fascia of the external abdominal oblique (Ext. oblique) and rectus abdominis (Rect. abdom.) muscles on each side of the linea alba. The preputial muscle is identified and sharply transected or cut with electrocautery, allowing retraction of the prepuce to the assistant side and further dissection and exposure of the linea. A stab incision is made into the linea alba, while elevating the linea. The incision is lengthened cranially and caudally either with scissors or using a blade and groove director.

Atlas of Surgical Approaches to Soft Tissue and Oncologic Diseases in the Dog and Cat, First Edition. Marije Risselada.
© 2020 John Wiley & Sons, Inc. Published 2020 by John Wiley & Sons, Inc.

Midline Approach to the Abdomen (Male Dog)

I)

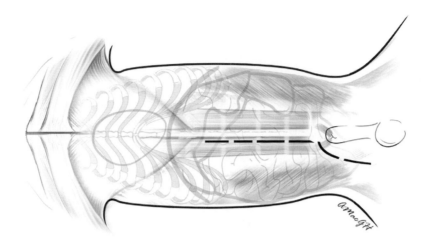

II)

Ext. oblique

Rect. abdom.

Prepucial m.

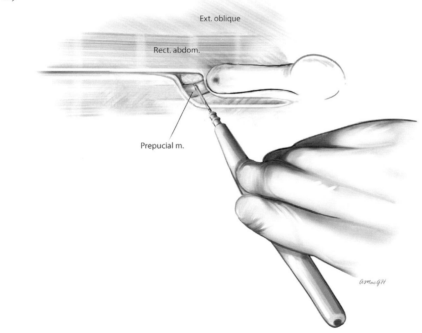

III)

Linea alba

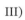

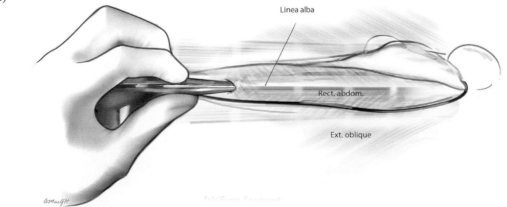

Rect. abdom.

Ext. oblique

PATIENT POSITIONING AND DESCRIPTION OF THE PROCEDURE *continued*

IV) Cranially the falciform ligament is seen. This can be either removed or reflected to the non-surgeon side. The liver (LV), intestines, and omentum are shown for illustrative purposes.

CLOSURE

Both sides of the incision are approximated, taking deep bites of the fascia and the linea and avoiding full thickness bites or incorporation of the peritoneal layer. The transected ends of the preputial muscle are reapposed. The remainder of the closure is routine and involves a subcutaneous layer, skin closure, with/without a deeper layer as needed based on body conformation/condition. The subcutaneous layer(s) can incorporate bites to the fascial layer, eliminating/minimizing dead space if desired.

ALTERNATE POSITIONING AND APPROACHES

- The skin incision can extend from the xiphoid to the pubis or can center only on the cranial or caudal abdomen.
- If needed, more access can be obtained by adding a caudal median sternotomy or a paracostal approach.
- The parapreputial incision can be either right- or left-sided, according to the handedness of the surgeon (right- or left-handed, respectively) or the presence of lesions.

Midline Approach to the Abdomen (Male Dog) *continued*

IV)

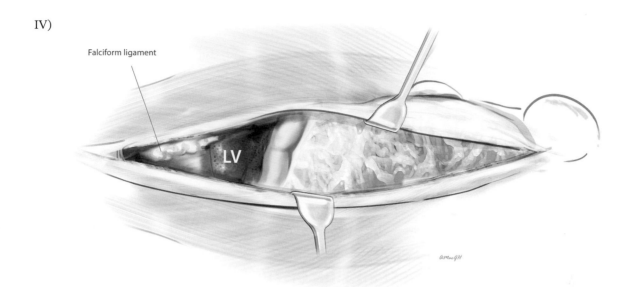

Falciform ligament

LV

Grid Approach to the Abdomen[8,17,25]

INDICATIONS

- Gastropexy (right side)
- G-tube placement (left side)

PATIENT POSITIONING AND DESCRIPTION OF THE PROCEDURE

I) The patient is placed in lateral recumbency with the lateral abdomen and caudal thorax clipped, prepped, and draped (or more as needed for the additional procedures). The skin incision is planned 5–10 cm caudal to the costal arch, in the ventral half of the lateral abdomen.

II) The subcutaneous tissues are dissected away from the fascia of the external abdominal oblique muscles. The muscle is split along the muscle fibers and retracted, exposing the internal abdominal oblique muscle. The internal abdominal oblique muscle is similarly split and retracted, revealing the transverse abdominis muscle, which is also split and retracted. This allows access to the abdomen.

CLOSURE

This is performed by apposing the three muscles individually, after which the subcutaneous tissues and skin are closed routinely.

ALTERNATE POSITIONING AND APPROACHES

- The patient can be placed in dorsal recumbency with the ventral abdomen clipped and prepped from cranial to the xyphoid to caudal to the pubis, extending dorsally to mid-abdomen on the left and right side (higher on the side of the intended approach).
- If a G-tube is placed, it is ideally tunneled through a separate incision, allowing the larger grid incision to heal.
- For a gastropexy, the seromuscular layer of the gastric wall is sutured to the transverse abdominis, after which the remainder of the closure is described as above.

Atlas of Surgical Approaches to Soft Tissue and Oncologic Diseases in the Dog and Cat, First Edition. Marije Risselada.
© 2020 John Wiley & Sons, Inc. Published 2020 by John Wiley & Sons, Inc.

Grid Approach to the Abdomen

I)

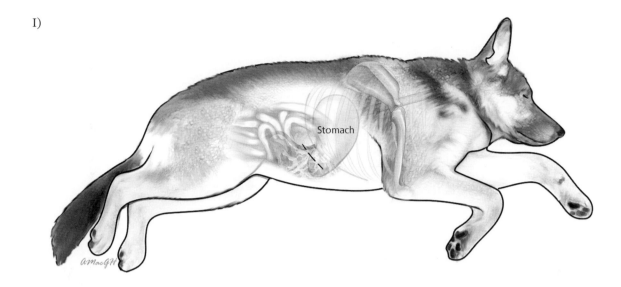

II)

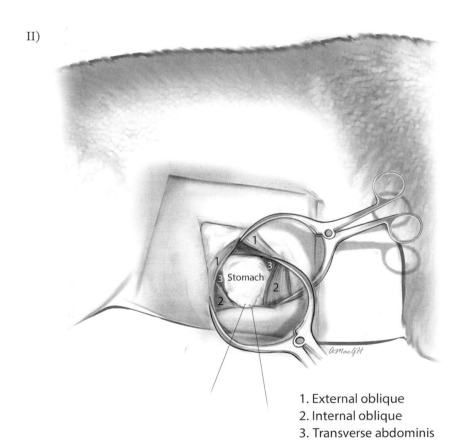

1. External oblique
2. Internal oblique
3. Transverse abdominis

Lateral Approach to the Dorsal Abdomen[3,17]

INDICATIONS

- Approach to the kidney, adrenal, or ovary unilaterally

PATIENT POSITIONING AND DESCRIPTION OF THE PROCEDURE

I) The lateral abdomen and lateral caudal thorax are clipped, from dorsal to the spinous processes to across the sternum/ventral midline. The patient is placed in lateral recumbency and the appropriate area is prepped and draped (or more as needed for the additional procedures). The skin incision is planned ventral to the lumbar spine, midway between the iliac wing and costal arch.

II, III) The subcutaneous tissues are dissected away from the fascia of the external abdominal oblique muscles. The muscle is split along the muscle fibers and retracted, exposing the internal abdominal oblique muscle. The internal abdominal oblique muscle is similarly split and retracted, revealing the transverse abdominis muscle, which is also split and retracted. This allows access to the abdomen.

Atlas of Surgical Approaches to Soft Tissue and Oncologic Diseases in the Dog and Cat, First Edition. Marije Risselada.
© 2020 John Wiley & Sons, Inc. Published 2020 by John Wiley & Sons, Inc.

Lateral Approach to the Dorsal Abdomen

I)

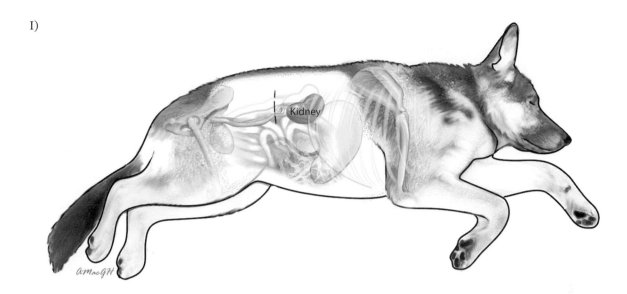

II)

1. External oblique
2. Internal oblique
3. Transverse abdominis

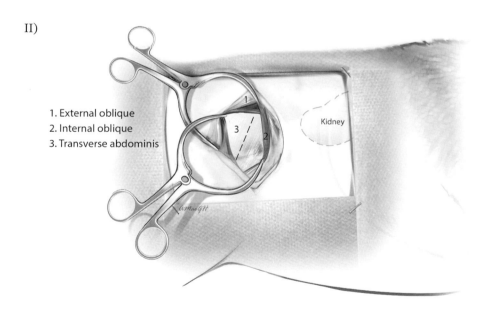

PATIENT POSITIONING AND DESCRIPTION OF THE PROCEDURE *continued*

II, III) The subcutaneous tissues are dissected away from the fascia of the external abdominal oblique muscles. The muscle is split along the muscle fibers and retracted, exposing the internal abdominal oblique muscle. The internal abdominal oblique muscle is similarly split and retracted, revealing the transverse abdominis muscle, which is also split and retracted. This allows access to the abdomen.

CLOSURE

This is performed by apposing the three muscles individually, after which the subcutaneous tissues and skin are closed routinely.

ALTERNATE POSITIONING AND APPROACHES

• A ventral midline allows access to all intraabdominal organs and, especially for full exploratory surgery or bilateral procedures, would be an appropriate approach.

Lateral Approach to the Dorsal Abdomen *continued*

III)

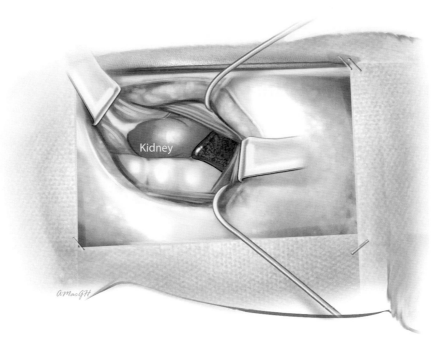

Paramedian Approach to the Inguinal Canal and Lymph Node[3,10,17]

INDICATIONS

- Extraabdominal inguinal herniorrhaphy
- Inguinal lymph node resection

PATIENT POSITIONING AND DESCRIPTION OF THE PROCEDURE

I, II) The patient is placed in dorsal recumbency with the ventral abdomen and cranial part of the pelvis clipped, prepped, and draped (or more as needed for the additional procedures). The skin incision is centered over the affected side, off midline.

Atlas of Surgical Approaches to Soft Tissue and Oncologic Diseases in the Dog and Cat, First Edition. Marije Risselada.
© 2020 John Wiley & Sons, Inc. Published 2020 by John Wiley & Sons, Inc.

Paramedian Approach to the Inguinal Canal and Lymph Node

I) Female

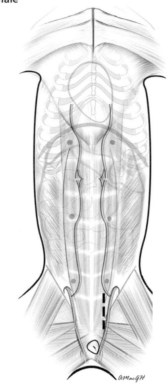

II) Male

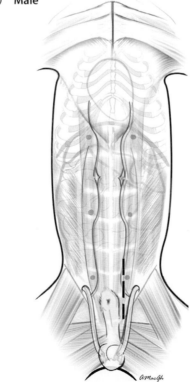

PATIENT POSITIONING AND DESCRIPTION OF THE PROCEDURE *continued*

III) The subcutaneous tissues are dissected away from the fascia of the external abdominal oblique muscles to identify either the inguinal lymph node (embedded in fat) or the inguinal hernia.

The inguinal canal consists of the external inguinal ring (an opening in the external abdominal oblique muscle and its tendon) and internal inguinal ring (rectus abdominis and internal abdominis oblique muscle and inguinal ligament). The hernial sac is identified and the contents are reduced into the abdomen if possible – the inguinal canal might need to be enlarged.

CLOSURE

In neutered males and in females, the canal is closed extraabdominally using an approximating pattern (simple interrupted or continuous), taking care not to strangulate the neurovascular bundle (external pudendal vessel, genital branch of the genitofemoral artery, vein, and nerve) at its caudal aspect. In intact male dogs the spermatic cord passes through the inguinal canal to the scrotum and care is taken not to strangulate it while closing the hernia.

ALTERNATE POSITIONING AND APPROACHES

- In bilateral inguinal hernias a midline skin incision can be performed with additional undermining and retraction to expose both inguinal canals individually.

Paramedian Approach to the Inguinal Canal and Lymph Node *continued*

III)

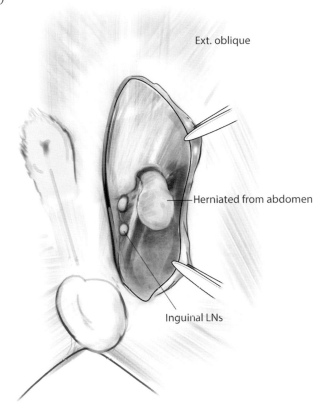

Ext. oblique

Herniated from abdomen

Inguinal LNs

Paracostal Approach to the Abdomen[3,17,25]

INDICATIONS

- Mesenteric lymph node access for lymphangiogram
- Approach to the cisterna chyli and thoracic duct

PATIENT POSITIONING AND DESCRIPTION OF THE PROCEDURE

I)   The lateral thorax and abdomen are clipped from dorsal (extending contralaterally) to ventral (extending to beyond midline/sternum). The patient is placed in lateral recumbency – a towel can be placed under the cranial abdomen if exposure to the thoracic duct is needed[26] and the patient prepped and draped (or more as needed for the additional procedures). The skin incision is planned along the right costal arch.

II) The subcutaneous tissues are dissected away from the fascia of the external abdominal oblique muscles. The abdominal muscles are transected along the line of the planned paracostal incision, taking care to leave enough muscles cranially for suturing.

CLOSURE

The paracostal incision is closed by reapposing the layers of the abdominal wall (full thickness), incorporating the rib if needed.

ALTERNATE POSITIONING AND APPROACHES

- The procedure is described for a right-sided paracostal approach.
- The abdominal wall muscles either can be sutured in a single layer if a single stage transection was performed or the different muscles can be reapposed individually if a grid-like exposure was used.
- *For exposure of the thorax*: the diaphragm is incised to gain access to the thoracic duct.[25] This incision is closed first, and negative intrathoracic pressure is established prior to abdominal wall closure.

Atlas of Surgical Approaches to Soft Tissue and Oncologic Diseases in the Dog and Cat, First Edition. Marije Risselada.
© 2020 John Wiley & Sons, Inc. Published 2020 by John Wiley & Sons, Inc.

Paracostal Approach to the Abdomen

I)

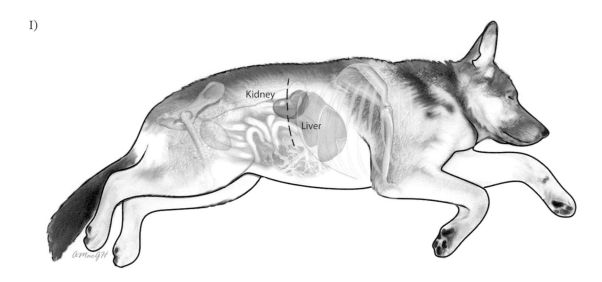

II)

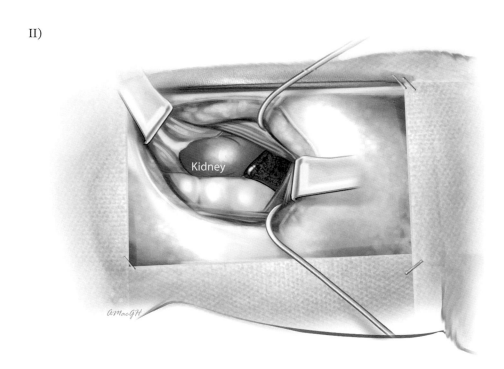

Combined Paracostal and Midline Approach to the Abdomen[3,17]

INDICATIONS

- Increased dorsolateral exposure for adrenal or liver tumors

PATIENT POSITIONING AND DESCRIPTION OF THE PROCEDURE

I)   The abdomen is clipped and prepped from cranial to the xiphoid to caudal to the pubis, extending dorsally to mid-abdomen on the left and right side – up to the spine on the side of the planned paracostal incision. The patient is placed in dorsal recumbency, aseptically prepared, and draped. The skin incision is planned along the midline and the right costal arch. Care is taken to not make the tip of the incision too acute in order to avoid a thin skin and muscle edge. The midline portion of the incision (1) is made prior to making the extension into the paracostal (2) incision.

II) The subcutaneous tissues are dissected away from the fascia of the external abdominal oblique (Ext. oblique) and rectus abdominis (Rect. abdom.) muscles on each side of the linea alba, extending to the end of the paracostal skin incision. A stab incision is made into the linea alba, while elevating the linea. The incision is lengthened cranially and caudally either with scissors or using a blade and groove director.

Atlas of Surgical Approaches to Soft Tissue and Oncologic Diseases in the Dog and Cat, First Edition. Marije Risselada.
© 2020 John Wiley & Sons, Inc. Published 2020 by John Wiley & Sons, Inc.

Combined Paracostal and Midline Approach to the Abdomen

I)

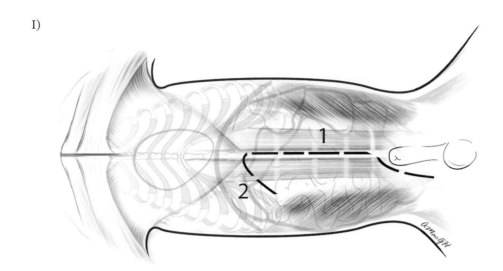

II)

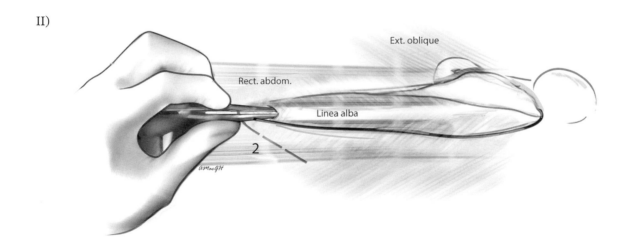

PATIENT POSITIONING AND DESCRIPTION OF THE PROCEDURE *continued*

III) The abdominal muscles are transected along the line of the planned paracostal incision, starting at midline, taking care to leave enough muscles cranially for suturing. The rectus abdominis (Rectus abdom.) is shown transected in the figure.

IV) The tip (where the two incisions join) is reattached in the appropriate corner in order to align all the wound edges appropriately. The paracostal incision is sutured first, with full thickness sutures reattaching the body wall, after which the midline incision is closed.

CLOSURE

Both sides of the incision are approximated, taking deep bites of the fascia and the linea, and avoiding full thickness bites or incorporation of the peritoneal layer. The subcutaneous tissues and skin are closed routinely.

ALTERNATE POSITIONING AND APPROACHES

- The procedure is described for a right-sided paracostal approach.
- The abdominal wall muscles either can be sutured in a single layer if a single stage transection was performed or the different muscles can be reapposed individually if a grid-like exposure was used.

Combined Paracostal and Midline Approach to the Abdomen *continued*

III)

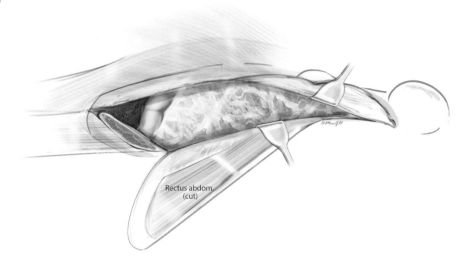

Rectus abdom.
(cut)

IV)

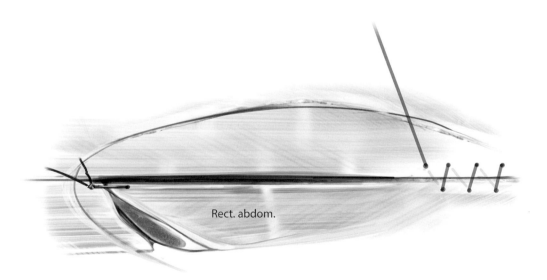

Rect. abdom.

Closure of a Caudal Abdominal Defect with Mesh[10,27]

INDICATIONS

- Prepubic tendon avulsion/rupture

PATIENT POSITIONING AND DESCRIPTION OF THE PROCEDURE

I) The ventral abdomen, from the caudal thorax to the pelvis, is clipped and prepped. The patient is placed in dorsal recumbency with the hind legs pulled back, but with the option to loosen the legs during the procedure to alleviate tension on the abdominal wall closure. The entire ventral abdomen is draped. The skin incision is planned along the midline.

II) The subcutaneous tissues are dissected away from the fascia of the external abdominal oblique muscles on each side of the linea alba and the cranial part of the pubis. Care is taken with any herniated abdominal contents or while breaking down adhesions in a more chronic abdominal wall hernia. The abdomen is entered routinely more cranial on midline if abdominal exploratory surgery is needed.

Atlas of Surgical Approaches to Soft Tissue and Oncologic Diseases in the Dog and Cat, First Edition. Marije Risselada.
© 2020 John Wiley & Sons, Inc. Published 2020 by John Wiley & Sons, Inc.

Closure of a Caudal Abdominal Defect with Mesh

I)

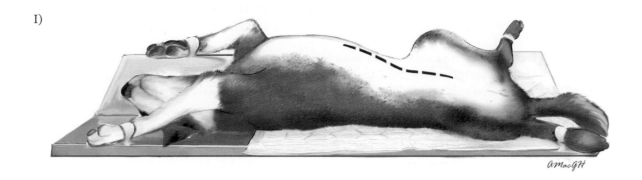

II)

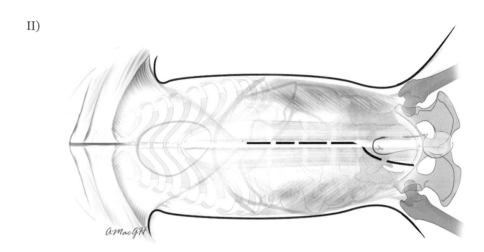

PATIENT POSITIONING AND DESCRIPTION OF THE PROCEDURE *continued*

III) Bone tunnels are drilled through the cranial rim of the pubic bone. The midline abdominal incision is closed first. If possible the abdominal wall is primarily reattached to the bone using heavy non-absorbable sutures and the predrilled bone tunnels.

IV) If there is too much tension for primary repair, mesh can be used to reconstruct the abdominal wall. Mesh is placed in the defect and attached to the pubic bone using heavy non-absorbable sutures and the bone tunnels. The abdominal wall is pulled under tension towards caudal and the mesh pulled flat in a cranial direction, allowing appropriate alignment of the abdominal wall with the mesh. The sutures attaching the mesh to the abdominal wall can be preplaced and then tied or they can be placed and tied individually. The remainder of the closure is routine.

ALTERNATE POSITIONING AND APPROACHES

- The edges of the mesh can either be laid flat or doubled over to avoid rubbing on and traumatizing the subcutaneous tissues and skin.

Closure of a Caudal Abdominal Defect with Mesh *continued*

III)

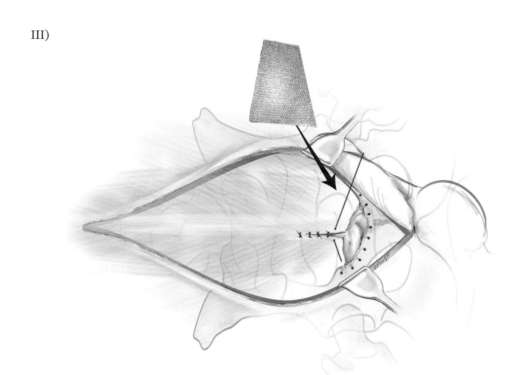

IV)

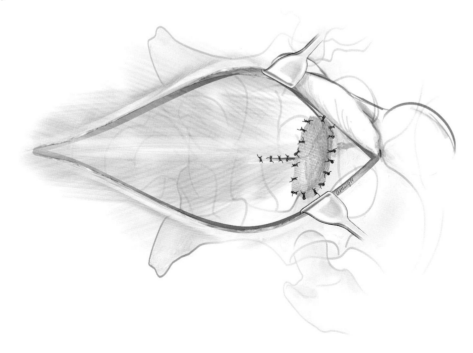

Approach to the Prescrotal Urethra[3]

INDICATIONS

- Prescrotal urethro(s)tomy

PATIENT POSITIONING AND DESCRIPTION OF THE PROCEDURE

I) The caudal abdomen, pelvic region, and perineal area are clipped and prepped. The patient is placed in dorsal recumbency with the hind legs extended and draped. The incision is planned in midline, over the median raphe, caudal to the os penis and cranial to the scrotum.

II) The subcutaneous tissues are bluntly dissected away to expose the penile tissues. The penis is manually stabilized to avoid rotation and to allow the retractor penis muscle to be identified. This muscle overlies the urethra and is bluntly dissected away and retracted.

Atlas of Surgical Approaches to Soft Tissue and Oncologic Diseases in the Dog and Cat, First Edition. Marije Risselada.

Approach to the Prescrotal Urethra

I)

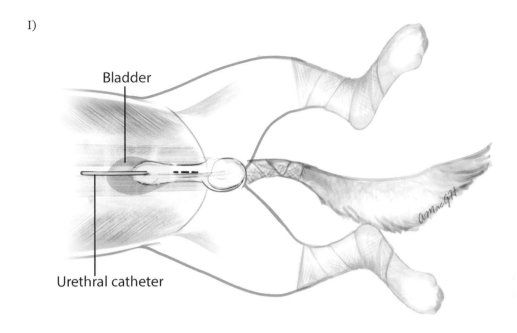

Bladder

Urethral catheter

II)

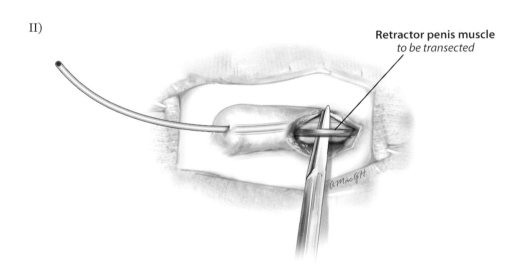

Retractor penis muscle
to be transected

PATIENT POSITIONING AND DESCRIPTION OF THE PROCEDURE *continued*

III) The urethra is identified by palpation and is entered via a stab incision. The urethrotomy is lengthened with straight iris scissors. The retractor penis muscle is either transected at the cranial and caudal border of the incision or pexied away (left or right from the incision.

CLOSURE

Closure of the urethrostomy is by apposing the urethral mucosa to the adjacent skin without tension. Closure is facilitated by approximating the deeper tissues first to alleviate tension on the urethrostomy closure.

ALTERNATE POSITIONING AND APPROACHES

- Placement of a urethral catheter facilitates palpation of the urethra and protects against inadvertent damage to the dorsal wall of the urethra.
- Ideally, the length of the urethrotomy should be 2–3 cm (based on the patient's size).
- Closure can be in simple interrupted sutures (absorbable or non-absorbable) or in a left and right simple continuous pattern (absorbable).
- Alternatively, a scrotal ablation and scrotal urethrostomy can be performed for recurrences or in small patients (as the scrotal urethra has a wider diameter than the prescrotal urethra).

Approach to the Prescrotal Urethra *continued*

III)

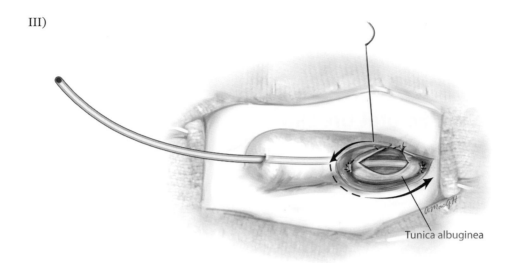

Tunica albuginea

Approach to the Scrotal Urethra[3]

INDICATIONS

- Scrotal urethrostomy

PATIENT POSITIONING AND DESCRIPTION OF THE PROCEDURE

I) The caudal abdomen, pelvic region, and perineal area are clipped and prepped. The patient is placed in dorsal recumbency with the hind legs extended and draped. The incision is similar to a scrotal ablation, taking care not to go too wide around the scrotal sac in order to avoid any tension on the urethrostomy.

II) A scrotal ablation neuter is performed first including neuter for intact dogs, after which the subcutaneous tissues are bluntly dissected away to expose the penile tissues. The penis is manually stabilized to avoid rotation and to allow the retractor penis muscle to be identified. This muscle overlies the urethra and is bluntly dissected away and retracted.

Approach to the Scrotal Urethra

I)

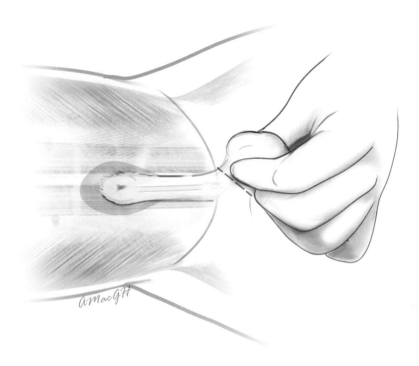

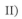

II)

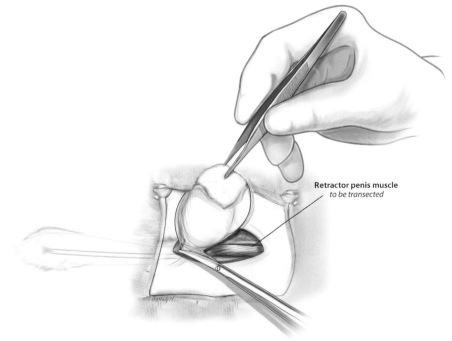

Retractor penis muscle
to be transected

PATIENT POSITIONING AND DESCRIPTION OF THE PROCEDURE *continued*

III) The urethra is identified by palpation and is entered via a stab incision. The urethrotomy is lengthened with straight iris scissors. The retractor penis muscle is either transected at the cranial and caudal border of the incision or pexied away (left or right from the incision).

CLOSURE

This is facilitated by approximating the deeper tissues first to alleviate tension on the urethrostomy closure. The urethrostomy closure is performed by apposing the urethral mucosa to the adjacent skin without tension.

ALTERNATE POSITIONING AND APPROACHES

- Placement of a urethral catheter facilitates palpation of the urethra and protects against inadvertent damage to the dorsal wall of the urethra.
- Ideally, the length of the urethrotomy should be 2–3 cm (based on the patient's size).
- Closure can be in simple interrupted sutures (absorbable or non-absorbable) or in a left and right simple continuous pattern (absorbable).
- Alternatively, a prescrotal urethrostomy or urethrotomy can be performed; however, the scrotal urethra has a wider diameter.

Approach to the Scrotal Urethra *continued*

III)

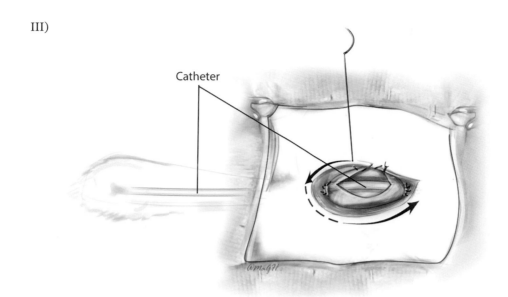

Catheter

Section 7

Perineal Area and Pelvic Canal

Dorsal Perineal Approach[3]

INDICATIONS

- Access to the caudal part of the pelvic canal – sacral lymph nodes, rectum

PATIENT POSITIONING AND DESCRIPTION OF THE PROCEDURE

I) The perineal area (extending laterally beyond the ischial tuberosity) including the base of the tail is clipped. The patient is placed in sternal recumbency in the Trendelenburg position, with the hindlimbs extending over the edge of the table and the tail pulled forward. A purse-string suture is placed in the anus. A curved incision is planned along the dorsal aspect of the anus/external anal sphincter.

II) The subcutaneous tissues are bluntly dissected along the external edge of the external anal sphincter to expose the rectococcygeal muscles.

Atlas of Surgical Approaches to Soft Tissue and Oncologic Diseases in the Dog and Cat, First Edition. Marije Risselada.
© 2020 John Wiley & Sons, Inc. Published 2020 by John Wiley & Sons, Inc.

Dorsal Perineal Approach

I)

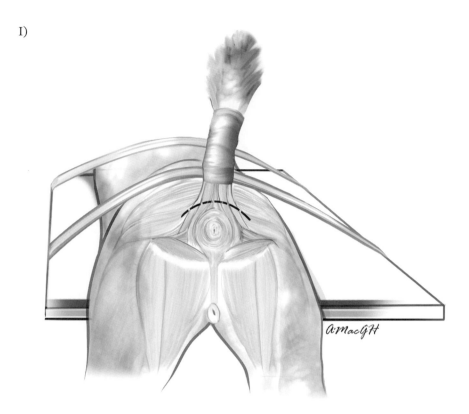

II)

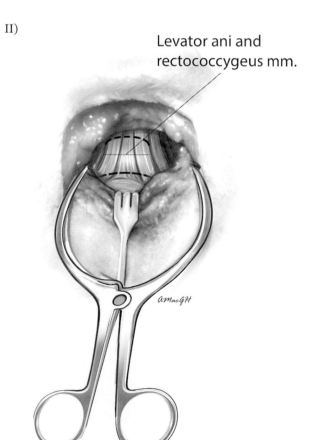

Levator ani and
rectococcygeus mm.

PATIENT POSITIONING AND DESCRIPTION OF THE PROCEDURE *continued*

III)   The rectococcygeal muscles are identified and transected to allow access to the dorsal part of the rectal canal.

CLOSURE

The transected muscles are reapposed first, followed by routine closure of the subcutaneous tissues and skin.

ALTERNATE POSITIONING AND APPROACHES

- Depending on the location of the lesion, this approach can be combined with a lateral approach to the perineal area.

Dorsal Perineal Approach *continued*

III)

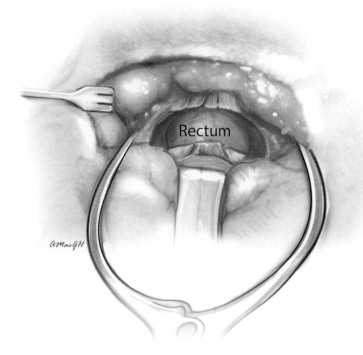

Lateral Perineal Approach for Perineal Hernia[1,3]

INDICATIONS

- Perineal hernia repair

PATIENT POSITIONING AND DESCRIPTION OF THE PROCEDURE

I) The perineal area (extending laterally beyond the ischial tuberosity) including the base of the tail is clipped. The patient is placed in sternal recumbency in the Trendelenburg position, with the hindlimbs extending over the edge of the table and the tail pulled forward. An anal purse-string suture is placed prior to prepping the case. The entire perineum is draped in for a bilateral procedure or only one side is draped in with the anus covered for a unilateral procedure. A curvilinear incision is planned lateral to the external anal sphincter, extending from the base of the tail to ventral to the ischium.

II) The hernia sac is identified, opened, and the contents are either reduced into the abdomen or amputated (strangulated fat). The perineal structures (external anal sphincter, levator ani, coccygeus and internal obturator muscles, as well as the sacrotuberous ligament and pudendal nerve) are identified.

The caudal ischial periosteal attachment of the internal obturator muscle is sharply incised, after which the muscle is elevated off the bone. The craniolateral tendon can be transected to allow better dorsomedial coverage.

Atlas of Surgical Approaches to Soft Tissue and Oncologic Diseases in the Dog and Cat, First Edition. Marije Risselada.
© 2020 John Wiley & Sons, Inc. Published 2020 by John Wiley & Sons, Inc.

Lateral Perineal Approach for Perineal Hernia

I)

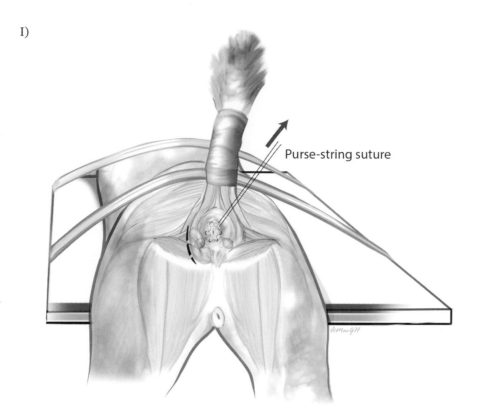

Purse-string suture

II)

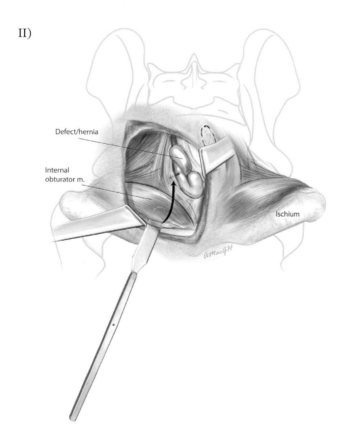

Defect/hernia

Internal
obturator m.

Ischium

PATIENT POSITIONING AND DESCRIPTION OF THE PROCEDURE *continued*

III) The internal obturator (IO) muscle is sutured in place to the external anal sphincter, the (remnants of the) levator ani and coccygeus muscles, if present, or the sacrotuberous ligament, taking care not to entrap the sciatic nerve on the cranial border of the ligament. The sutures are preplaced and then tied while keeping traction on the other preplaced sutures.

CLOSURE

The perineal diaphragm is reconstructed using preplaced sutures (see above in section III). The remainder of the closure is routine.

ALTERNATE POSITIONING AND APPROACHES

- The incision can be angled in a dorsomedial to ventrolateral direction to allow better lateral access distally/ventrally.
- This approach can also be used for access to lateral perineal tumors, with separation of the muscles of the pelvic diaphragm and subsequent reapposition upon closure.

Lateral Perineal Approach for Perineal Hernia *continued*

III)

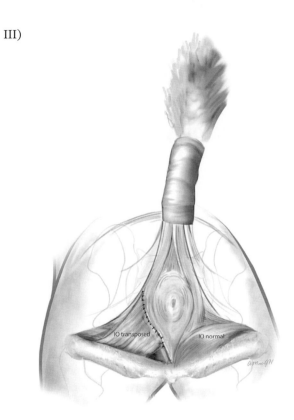

Approach for Anal Sacculectomy[1]

INDICATIONS

- Closed approach for anal sacculectomy and anal sac tumor removals
- Open approach for anal sacculectomy

PATIENT POSITIONING AND DESCRIPTION OF THE PROCEDURE

I)   The perineal area (extending laterally beyond the ischial tuberosity) including the base of the tail is clipped. The patient is placed in sternal recumbency in the Trendelenburg position, with the hindlimbs extending over the edge of the table and the tail pulled forward. An anal purse-string suture is placed prior to prepping the case, taking care to leave the orifice of the anal sac duct superficial to the purse-string.

   The entire perineum is draped in for a bilateral procedure or only one side is draped in with the anus covered for a unilateral procedure. A curvilinear incision is planned lateral to the external anal sphincter centered over the anal sac (5 and 7 o'clock).

II) The subcutaneous tissues are dissected off the anal sac (tumor). The anal sac and its duct lie embedded in the external anal sphincter. The muscle fibers are bluntly dissected off the sac, staying close to the tumor/anal sac. The duct is either ligated close to its orifice or it is transected at the level of the orifice, after which the resulting defect is closed with one or two simple interrupted buried sutures.

CLOSURE

The deeper layers (including the muscles of the external anal sphincter) are approximated and apposed. The subcutaneous layers and skin are closed routinely.

ALTERNATE POSITIONING AND APPROACHES

- *Open approach*: an alternate approach for anal sacculectomy is to place a groove director into the duct and anal sac and transect all overlying structures from the ductal orifice to the lateral-most aspect of the anal sac. The anal sac is dissected out from the duct to the lateral-most aspect, the wound bed flushed, and the external anal sphincter muscle is reapposed prior to closing the remaining layers routinely.

Atlas of Surgical Approaches to Soft Tissue and Oncologic Diseases in the Dog and Cat, First Edition. Marije Risselada.
© 2020 John Wiley & Sons, Inc. Published 2020 by John Wiley & Sons, Inc.

Approach for Anal Sacculectomy

I)

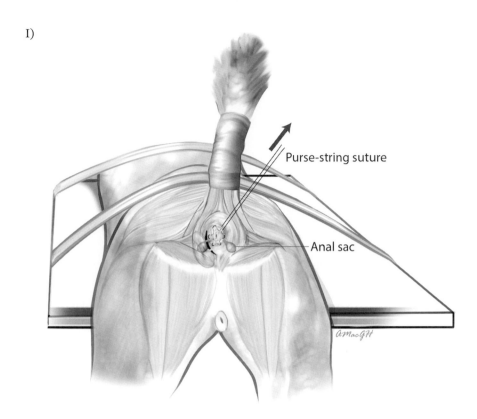

Purse-string suture

Anal sac

II)

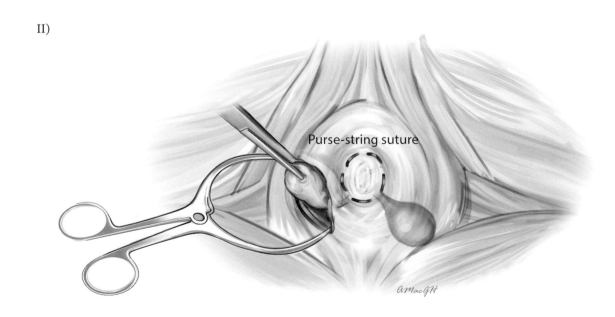

Purse-string suture

Episiotomy[3]

INDICATIONS

- Access to the vestibulum and vagina.

PATIENT POSITIONING AND DESCRIPTION OF THE PROCEDURE

I)   The perineal area (extending laterally beyond the ischial tuberosity) including the base of the tail is clipped. The patient is placed in sternal recumbency in the Trendelenburg position, with the hindlimbs extending over the edge of the table and the tail pulled forward. A skin incision is planned along midline (median raphe).

II) The muscles are transected along the line of the skin incision, as is the mucosa. A stay suture can be placed in the free (ventral) edge of the incision to facilitate manipulation.

Atlas of Surgical Approaches to Soft Tissue and Oncologic Diseases in the Dog and Cat, First Edition. Marije Risselada.
© 2020 John Wiley & Sons, Inc. Published 2020 by John Wiley & Sons, Inc.

Episiotomy

I)

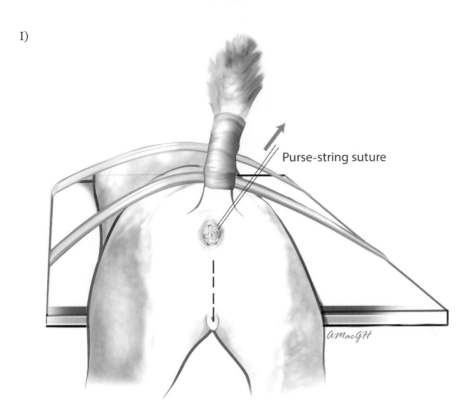

Purse-string suture

II)

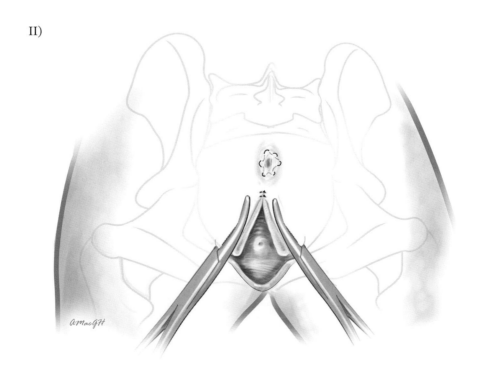

CLOSURE

III, IV)   A three-layer closure is performed: the mucosal layer is sutured first (1) (in a simple continuous or simple interrupted pattern), allowing the knots to be buried within the tissue. The muscle layer is closed next (2) in a separate layer, and the skin is closed routinely (3). A subcutaneous layer can be added if needed.

ALTERNATE POSITIONING AND APPROACHES

- If excessive bleeding is encountered, non-crushing or intestinal forceps can be placed on either side of the incision to temporarily occlude vessels.
- A urinary catheter can be placed during the procedure to allow identification of the urethra during dissection.

Episiotomy *continued*

III)

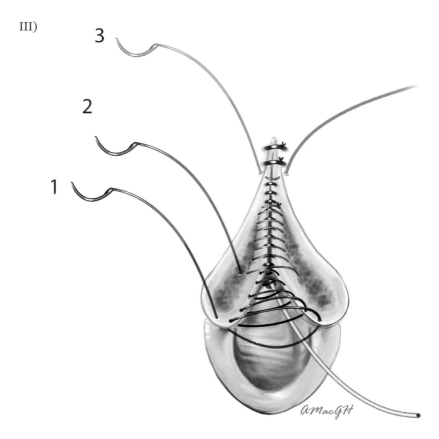

IV)

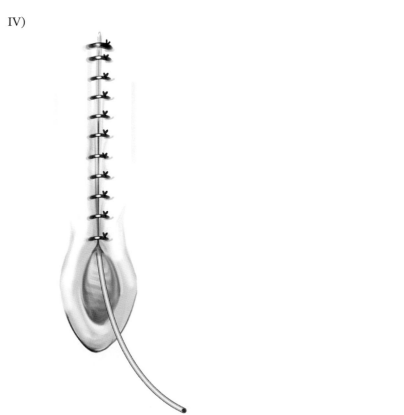

Approach for Feline Perineal Urethrostomy[1,3,8]

INDICATIONS

- Perineal urethrostomy

PATIENT POSITIONING AND DESCRIPTION OF THE PROCEDURE

I) The perineal area (extending laterally beyond the ischial tuberosity) including the base of the tail is clipped. The patient is placed in sternal recumbency in the Trendelenburg position, with the hindlimbs extending over the edge of the table and the tail pulled forward.

II) A purse-string suture is placed in the anus and the entire perineum is clipped, prepped, and draped. An elliptical incision is planned around the scrotum and prepuce.

Atlas of Surgical Approaches to Soft Tissue and Oncologic Diseases in the Dog and Cat, First Edition. Marije Risselada.
© 2020 John Wiley & Sons, Inc. Published 2020 by John Wiley & Sons, Inc.

Approach for Feline Perineal Urethrostomy

I)

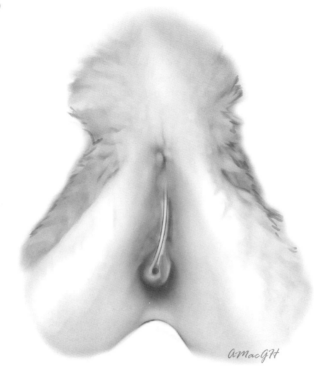

II)

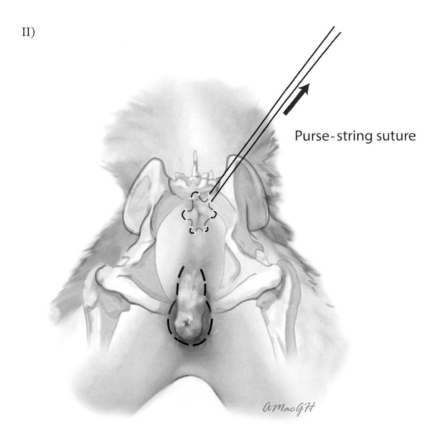

Purse-string suture

PATIENT POSITIONING AND DESCRIPTION OF THE PROCEDURE *continued*

III) The subcutaneous tissues are dissected off the penile tissues, freeing it up from its distal and ventral attachments. Dissection is continued cranially ventral to the penis to expose the ischiocavernosus muscles. These muscles are transected along their periosteal attachment bilaterally and elevated off the ischial bone. Any remaining fibrous tissue attachments ventrally are bluntly broken down, allowing visualization of the bulbourethral glands. The planned urethrostomy site extends cranial to the bulbourethral glands. The retractor penis muscle is dissected off the surface of the urethra. A stab incision is made in the urethra (ideally with a urethral catheter in place to avoid damaging the opposite side of the urethra) and lengthened using straight microdissection scissors or iris scissors.

Approach for Feline Perineal Urethrostomy *continued*

III)

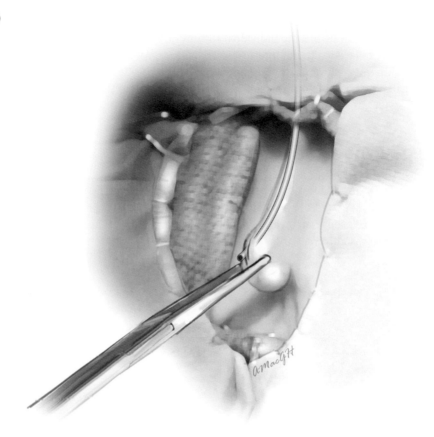

PATIENT POSITIONING AND DESCRIPTION OF THE PROCEDURE *continued*

IV, V) Closure of the urethrostomy is started by placing a suture from the skin to the urethral mucosa at the 11 and 1 o'clock positions. The remaining penile urethra is used as a drain board and the urethral mucosa is sutured to the skin. This can be done either by placing individual sutures or by closing each side as a simple continuous pattern, using the initial sutures placed at the 11 and 1 o'clock positions. An additional suture can be placed in a triangular pattern, engaging skin–mucosa–skin at the 12 o'clock position if needed.

The penis is ligated distal to the drain board and transected distal to the ligature, after which the ventral skin is closed routinely.

ALTERNATE POSITIONING AND APPROACHES

- An alternate approach is to position the animal in dorsal recumbency with the legs pulled forward and laterally, allowing simultaneous access to the bladder and the perineum, if cystotomy is needed.[27]
- Approximating sutures can be placed from the transected ischiocavernosus muscles to the subcutaneous tissues to relieve any tension on the urethrostomy closure.

Approach for Feline Perineal Urethrostomy *continued*

IV)

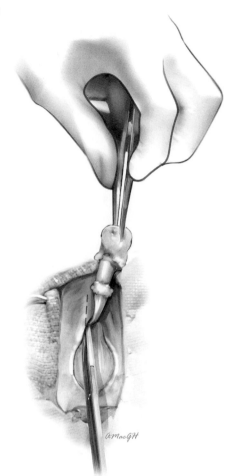

V)

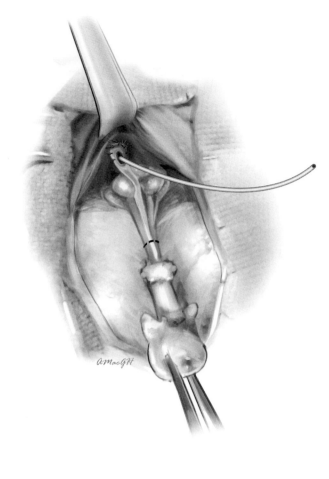

Ventral Approach to the Pelvic Canal[2,3,8]

INDICATIONS

- Intrapelvic tumors and lesions

PATIENT POSITIONING AND DESCRIPTION OF THE PROCEDURE

I)   The caudal abdomen, pelvic region, and perineal area are clipped and prepped. The patient is placed in dorsal recumbency with the hind legs extended with the abdomen, pelvic region, and perineal area draped.

II, III)   A midline incision is planned in female dogs and cats and a parapreputial incision is planned for male dogs.

The subcutaneous tissues and inguinal fat are bluntly dissected off the pubic bone and pelvic musculature (gracilis and adductor muscles ventrally and the prepubic tendon cranially). In male dogs the preputial muscle is transected and the blunt dissection is continued dorsal to the penis, until the penis can be retracted away from the pubic bone and pelvic musculature.

Atlas of Surgical Approaches to Soft Tissue and Oncologic Diseases in the Dog and Cat, First Edition. Marije Risselada.
© 2020 John Wiley & Sons, Inc. Published 2020 by John Wiley & Sons, Inc.

Ventral Approach to the Pelvic Canal

I)

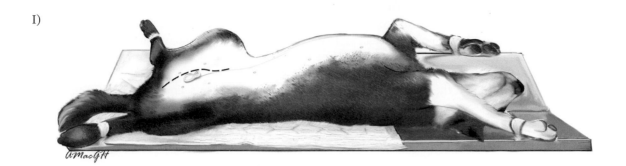

II)

III)

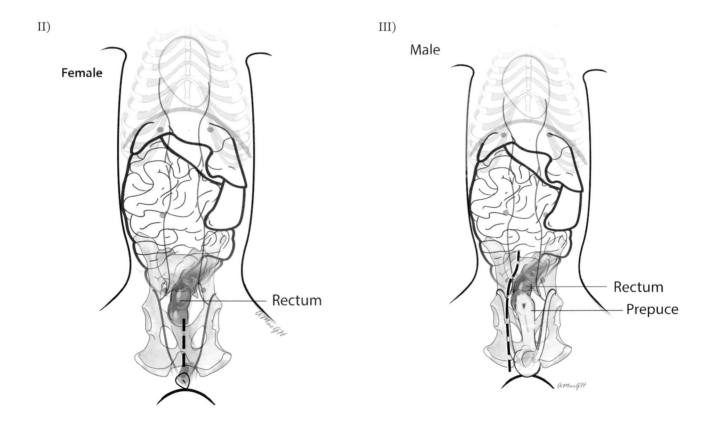

Female

Rectum

Male

Rectum

Prepuce

PATIENT POSITIONING AND DESCRIPTION OF THE PROCEDURE *continued*

IV) *Symphysectomy*: the pelvic muscles are elevated off the bone and the prepubic tendon is sharply transected at its periosteal attachment to expose the area of bone that will be removed. The intrapelvic organs are protected with a malleable retractor. Bone tunnels are drilled on the medial and lateral aspects of the osteotomy sites (allowing enough space) to facilitate reattachment post surgery. Additional bone tunnels are drilled along the cranial border to allow reattachment of the abdominal wall.

V) The osteotomies are completed and the bone segment is removed and wrapped in saline-soaked gauze until it is replaced during closure. Closure starts with reattaching the bone segment using cerclage wires and the predrilled bone tunnels, after which the abdominal wall is reattached to the bone using predrilled bone tunnels.

CLOSURE

The pelvic floor is restored first by reattaching the bone using predrilled bone tunnels. The abdominal wall is reattached to the bone using bone tunnels. The remainder of the closure is routine, taking care to avoid excessive dead space, especially in male dogs.

ALTERNATE POSITIONING AND APPROACHES

- In cats or small dogs, a pubic symphysiotomy can be performed and both bone edges retracted laterally using Gelpi retractors. The pelvic muscles are elevated off the symphysis, clearing enough space bilaterally for visualization of the bone tunnels. These can be drilled either prior to or after performing the symphysiotomy.
- If the bone cannot be replaced, the pelvic canal can be reconstructed by suturing non-absorbable mesh in its place using the predrilled bone tunnels.

Ventral Approach to the Pelvic Canal *continued*

IV)

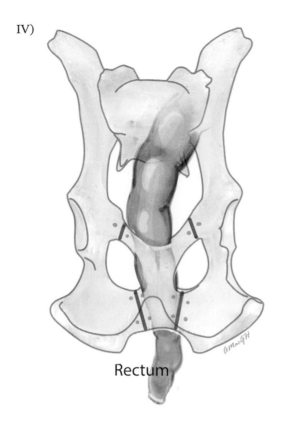

Rectum

V)

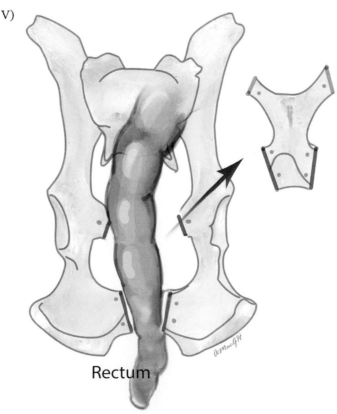

Rectum

Section 8

Digits and Tail

Lateral Approach to Digit 1[3,17]

INDICATIONS

- Digit amputations

PATIENT POSITIONING AND DESCRIPTION OF THE PROCEDURE

I) The distal areas of the limb, including all the digits, are clipped and prepped. The clipped area must extend proximal enough to allow adequate room to place a tourniquet and/or manipulation of the leg after draping.

Digit 1: the patient is placed in lateral recumbency with the affected leg down. The uppermost leg is pulled caudally (forelimb) or cranially (hindlimb) and the affected leg is positioned such that it extends beyond the edge of the table, allowing circumferential draping without necessitating a hanging limb draping technique. The planned incision is circumferential around digit 1.

Lateral Approach to Digit 1

I)

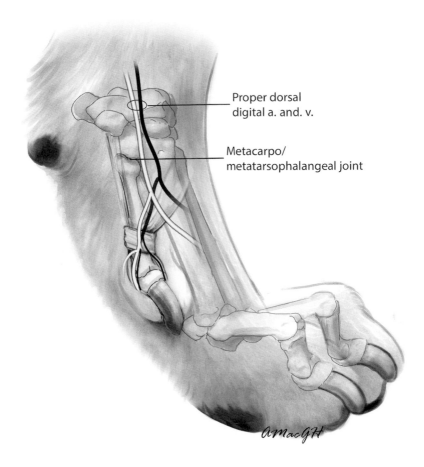

Proper dorsal
digital a. and. v.

Metacarpo/
metatarsophalangeal joint

PATIENT POSITIONING AND DESCRIPTION OF THE PROCEDURE *continued*

II) The subcutaneous tissues are dissected away bluntly and the metacarpo- or metatarsophalangeal joint is identified. The muscles are transected at their origins and the joint is disarticulated.

III) The deeper tissues are approximated first.

CLOSURE

The closure is routine.

ALTERNATE POSITIONING AND APPROACHES

- For a forelimb digital amputation, the patient can be placed in dorsal recumbency, especially if bilateral access is needed.
- The sesamoid bones caudal to the joint can be removed or left in situ.
- If desired, a lower (phalangeal–phalangeal) amputation can be performed using a similar technique.
- A tourniquet can be placed around the distal limb to decrease bleeding. Release of the tourniquet prior to closure allows for a check of hemostasis.

Lateral Approach to Digit 1 *continued*

II)

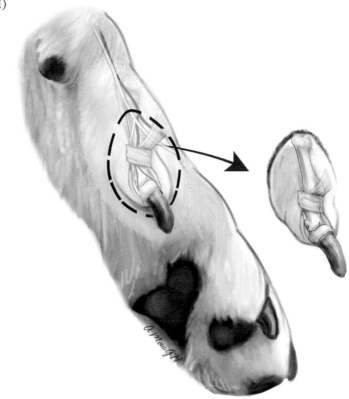

III)

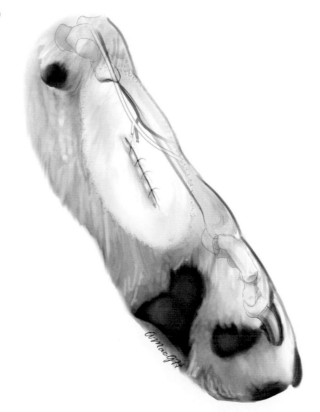

Lateral Approach to Digit 2[3,17]

INDICATIONS

- Digit amputations

PATIENT POSITIONING AND DESCRIPTION OF THE PROCEDURE

I) The distal areas of the limb, including all the digits, are clipped and prepped. The clipped area must extend proximal enough to allow adequate room to place a tourniquet and/or manipulation of the leg after draping.

  Digit 2: the patient is placed in lateral recumbency with the affected leg down. The uppermost leg is pulled caudally (forelimb) or cranially (hindlimb) and the affected leg is positioned such that it extends beyond the edge of the table, allowing circumferential draping without necessitating a hanging limb draping technique. The planned incision is teardrop shaped on the medial aspect of the leg (digit 2).

Atlas of Surgical Approaches to Soft Tissue and Oncologic Diseases in the Dog and Cat, First Edition. Marije Risselada.
© 2020 John Wiley & Sons, Inc. Published 2020 by John Wiley & Sons, Inc.

Lateral Approach to Digit 2

I)

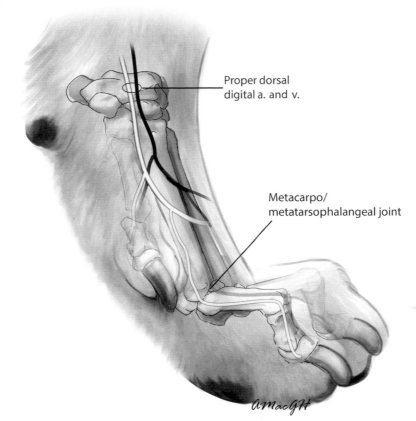

Proper dorsal
digital a. and v.

Metacarpo/
metatarsophalangeal joint

PATIENT POSITIONING AND DESCRIPTION OF THE PROCEDURE *continued*

II) The subcutaneous tissue are dissected away bluntly and the metacarpo- or metatarsophalangeal joint is identified. The muscles are transected at their origins and the joint is disarticulated.

III) The deeper tissues are approximated first.

CLOSURE

The closure is routine.

ALTERNATE POSITIONING AND APPROACHES

- The digit can be approached dorsally (see Dorsal Approach to Digit 5) instead of a laterally oriented approach.
- For a forelimb digital amputation, the patient can be placed in dorsal recumbency, especially if bilateral access is needed.
- The sesamoid bones caudal to the joint can be removed or left in situ.
- If desired, a lower (phalangeal–phalangeal) amputation can be performed using a similar technique.
- A tourniquet can be placed around the distal limb to decrease bleeding. Release of the tourniquet prior to closure allows for a check of hemostasis.

Lateral Approach to Digit 2 *continued*

II)

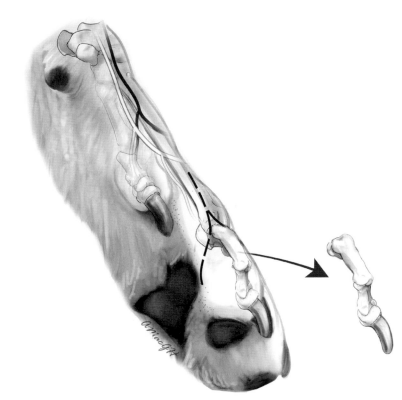

III)

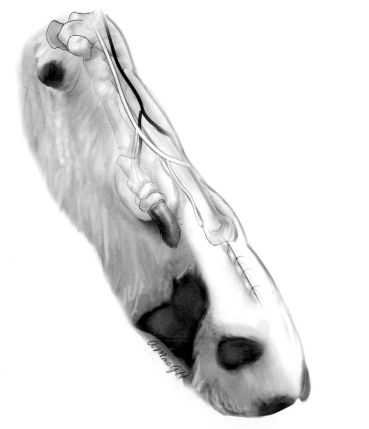

Dorsal Approach to Digits 3 and 4[2]

INDICATIONS

- Digit amputations

PATIENT POSITIONING AND DESCRIPTION OF THE PROCEDURE

I)   The patient is placed in dorsal recumbency with the affected leg uppermost and prepped using a hanging limb set-up. The planned incision is teardrop shaped.
II) The subcutaneous tissue are dissected away bluntly and the metacarpo-/metatarsophalangeal joint is identified. The muscles are transected at their origins and the joint is disarticulated.

Atlas of Surgical Approaches to Soft Tissue and Oncologic Diseases in the Dog and Cat, First Edition. Marije Risselada.
© 2020 John Wiley & Sons, Inc. Published 2020 by John Wiley & Sons, Inc.

Dorsal Approach to Digits 3 and 4

I)

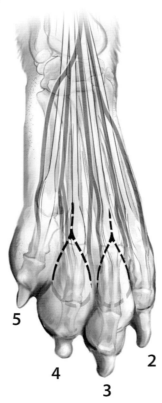

II)

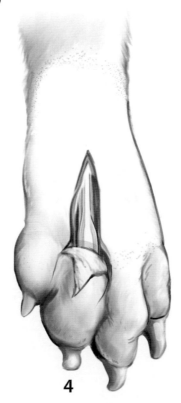

PATIENT POSITIONING AND DESCRIPTION OF THE PROCEDURE *continued*

III, IV)   The deeper tissues are approximated first. The medial and lateral portions of the skin incision can be apposed to create a new interdigital web; alternatively, if more skin was resected, the dorsal and palmar/plantar edges of each digit can be apposed separately.

Removal of the 3rd and 4th phalanx are shown in separate images.

CLOSURE

The closure is routine.

ALTERNATE POSITIONING AND APPROACHES

- Alternatively, a lateral or medial approach can be used.
- The sesamoid bones caudal to the joint can be removed or left in situ.
- If desired, a lower (phalangeal–phalangeal) amputation can be performed using a similar technique.
- If two digits are to be removed, the teardrop incision is outlined to incorporate both digits.

Dorsal Approach to Digits 3 and 4 *continued*

III)

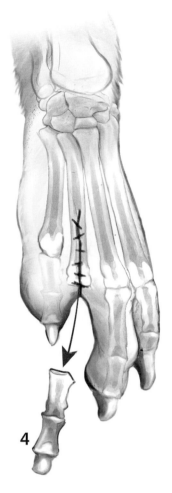

4

IV)

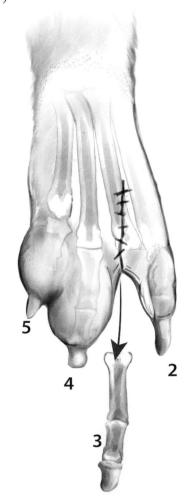

5

4

2

3

Dorsal Approach to Digit 5[3,17]

INDICATIONS

- Digit amputations

PATIENT POSITIONING AND DESCRIPTION OF THE PROCEDURE

I)   The distal areas of the limb, including all the digits, are clipped and prepped. The clipped area must extend proximal enough to allow adequate room to place a tourniquet and/or manipulation of the leg after draping.
     Digit 5: the patient is placed in lateral recumbency with the affected leg uppermost and prepped using a hanging limb set-up. The planned incision is teardrop shaped on the lateral aspect of the leg.

II) The subcutaneous tissues are dissected away bluntly and the metacarpo- or metatarsophalangeal joint is identified. The muscles are transected at their origins and the joint is disarticulated.

Atlas of Surgical Approaches to Soft Tissue and Oncologic Diseases in the Dog and Cat, First Edition. Marije Risselada.
© 2020 John Wiley & Sons, Inc. Published 2020 by John Wiley & Sons, Inc.

Dorsal Approach to Digit 5

I)

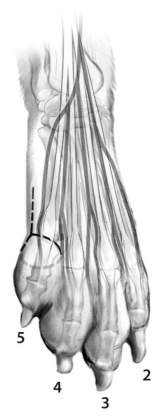

II)

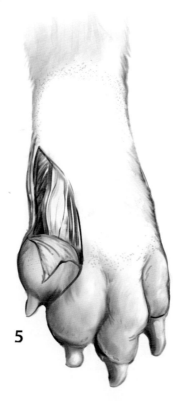

PATIENT POSITIONING AND DESCRIPTION OF THE PROCEDURE *continued*

III)   The deeper tissues are approximated first.

CLOSURE

The closure is routine.

ALTERNATE POSITIONING AND APPROACHES

- The digit can be approached laterally (see Lateral Approach to Digit 2) instead of a dorsally oriented approach.
- For a forelimb digital amputation, the patient can be placed in dorsal recumbency, especially if bilateral access is needed.
- The sesamoid bones caudal to the joint can be removed or left in situ.
- If desired, a lower (phalangeal–phalangeal) amputation can be performed using similar technique.
- A tourniquet can be placed around the distal limb to decrease bleeding. Release of the tourniquet prior to closure allows for a check of hemostasis.

Dorsal Approach to Digit 5 *continued*

III)

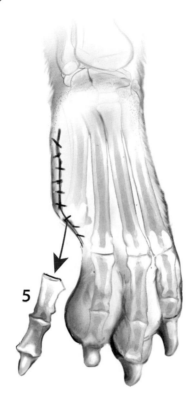

5

Dorsal Approach to the Sacrococcygeal Joint[1,13]

INDICATIONS

- Total caudectomy at the sacrococcygeal level

PATIENT POSITIONING AND DESCRIPTION OF THE PROCEDURE

I) The dorsal lumbar area, base of the tail, and the perineal areas (extending laterally beyond the ischial tuberosity) area clipped. The patient is placed in ventral recumbency with the tail suspended to allow a hanging limb draping technique. The incision is planned in an elliptical or teardrop shape around the tail base. The tip of the teardrop is towards the head of the patient, along the midline.

II) The muscles of the tail (sacrocaudalis dorsalis lateralis and medialis; sacrocaudalis ventralis lateralis and medialis; intertransversarius dorsalis and ventralis caudalis) are sharply transected and dissected away from the intervertebral space. Care is taken to provide adequate hemostasis (such as coagulation or ligation) for the arteries, including the median caudal, lateral caudal, and the dorsal and ventral lateral caudal arteries.

Atlas of Surgical Approaches to Soft Tissue and Oncologic Diseases in the Dog and Cat, First Edition. Marije Risselada.
© 2020 John Wiley & Sons, Inc. Published 2020 by John Wiley & Sons, Inc.

Dorsal Approach to the Sacrococcygeal Joint

I)

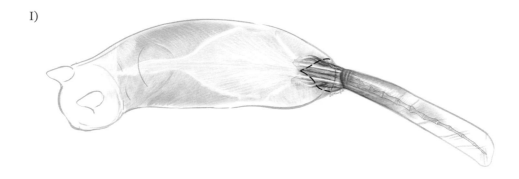

II)

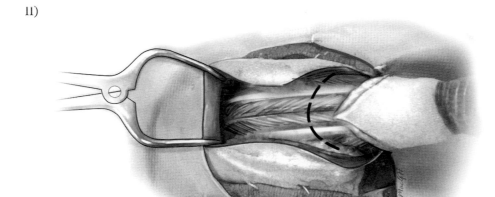

PATIENT POSITIONING AND DESCRIPTION OF THE PROCEDURE *continued*

III) The joint space is located and disarticulated with a blade or heavy scissors. The remaining cartilage at the proximal vertebra can be removed with rongeurs.

CLOSURE

IV) Closure is started with approximating sutures in the deeper tissues, followed by routine closure. The skin flaps can be trimmed if excess skin is present.

ALTERNATE POSITIONING AND APPROACHES

● For lower lesions, a coccygeal–coccygeal amputation is preferred over a sacrococcygeal amputation.

Dorsal Approach to the Sacrococcygeal Joint *continued*

III)

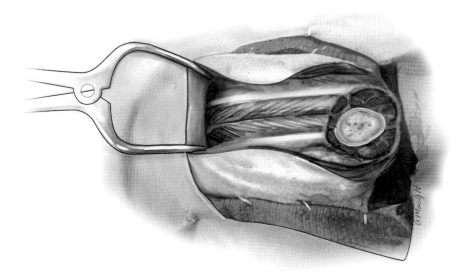

IV)

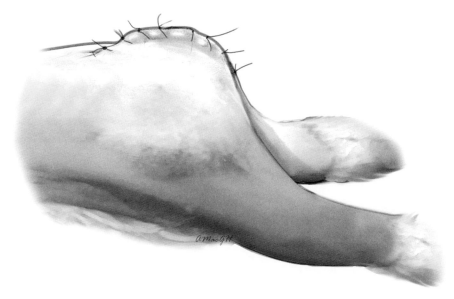

References

1 Caywood, D.D. and Lipowitz, A.J. (1989). *Atlas of General Small Animal Surgery*. St Louis, MO: C.V. Mosby Company.

2 Piermattei, D.L. and Johnson, K.A. (2004). *An Atlas of Surgical Approaches to the Bones and Joints of the Dog and Cat*, 4e. Philadelphia, PA: Saunders.

3 Smith, M.M. and Waldron, D.R. (1993). *Atlas of Approaches for General Surgery of the Dog and Cat*. Philadelphia, PA: W.B. Saunders.

4 Lascelles, B.D.X., Henderson, R.A., Seguin, B. et al. (2004). Bilateral rostral maxillectomy and nasal planectomy for large rostral maxillofacial neoplasms in six dogs and one cat. *Journal of the American Animal Hospital Association* 40: 137–146.

5 Gallegos, J., Schmiedt, C.W., and McAnulty, J.F. (2007). Cosmetic rostral nasal reconstruction after nasal planum and premaxilla resection: technique and results in two dogs. *Veterinary Surgery* 36: 669–674.

6 Tobias, K.M. and Johnston, S.A. (2013). *Veterinary Surgery: Small Animal*. Elsevier Health Sciences.

7 Ter Haar, G. and Hampel, R. (2015). Combined rostrolateral rhinotomy for removal of rostral nasal septum squamous cell carcinoma: long-term outcome in 10 dogs. *Veterinary Surgery* 44: 843–851.

8 Bojrab, M.J. (1997). *Current Techniques in Small Animal Surgery*, 4e. Baltimore, MD: Williams & Wilkins.

9 Lascelles, B.D.X., Thomson, M.J., Dernell, W.S. et al. (2003). Combined dorsolateral and intraoral approach for the resection of tumors of the maxilla in the dog. *Journal of the American Animal Hospital Association* 39: 294–305.

10 Slatter, D. (2003). *Textbook of Small Animal Surgery*, 3e. Philadelphia, PA: Saunders.

11 Mathews, K.G., Hardie, E.M., and Murphy, K.M. (2006). Subtotal ear canal ablation in 18 dogs and one cat with minimal distal ear canal pathology. *Journal of the American Animal Hospital Association* 42: 371–380.

12 Marsh, A. and Adin, C. (2013). Tunneling under the digastricus muscle increases salivary duct exposure and completeness of excision in mandibular and sublingual sialoadenectomy in dogs. *Veterinary Surgery* 42 (3): 238–242.

13 Ritter, M.J., von Pfeil, D.J.F., Stanley, B.J. et al. (2006). Mandibular and sublingual sialocoeles in the dog: a retrospective evaluation of 41 cases, using the ventral approach for treatment. *New Zealand Veterinary Journal* 54: 333–337.

14 Wright, T. and Oblak, M.K. (2016). Lymphadenectomy: overview of surgical anatomy & removal of peripheral lymph nodes. *Today's Veterinary Practice* (July/August), pp. 20–29.

15 Green, K. and Boston, S.E. (2015). Bilateral removal of the mandibular and medial retropharyngeal lymph nodes through a single ventral midline incision for staging of head and neck cancers in dogs: a description of surgical technique. *Veterinary and Comparative Oncology* 2015: 1–7.

16 Orton, E.C. (1995). *Small Animal Thoracic Surgery*. Malvern, PA: Williams & Wilkins.

17 Evans, H.E. (1993). *Miller's Anatomy of the Dog*, 3e. Philadelphia, PA: Saunders.

18 Norton, C., Drenen, C.M., and Emms, S.G. (2006). Subtotal scapulectomy as the treatment for scapular tumours in the dog: a report of six cases. *Australian Veterinary Journal* 84: 364–366.

19 Sharp, N.J.H. (1988). Craniolateral approach to the canine brachial plexus. *Veterinary Surgery* 17: 18–21.

20 Bray, J.P. (2014). Hemipelvectomy: modified surgical technique and clinical experiences from a retrospective study. *Veterinary Surgery* 43: 19–26.

21 Barbur, L.A., Coleman, K.D., Schmiedt, C.W. et al. (2015). Description of the anatomy, surgical technique, and outcome of hemipelvectomy in 4 dogs and 5 cats. *Veterinary Surgery* 44: 613–626.

22 Kramer, A., Walsh, P.J., and Seguin, B.H. (2008). Hemipelvectomy in dogs and cats: technique overview, variations, and description. *Veterinary Surgery* 37: 413–419.

Atlas of Surgical Approaches to Soft Tissue and Oncologic Diseases in the Dog and Cat, First Edition. Marije Risselada.
© 2020 John Wiley & Sons, Inc. Published 2020 by John Wiley & Sons, Inc.

23 Aronsohn, M. (1984). Diaphragmatic advancement for defects of the caudal thoracic wall in the dog. *Veterinary Surgery* 13: 26–28.

24 Visser, L.C., Keene, B.W., Mathews, K.G. et al. (2013). Outcomes and complications associated with epicardial pacemakers in 28 dogs and 5 cats. *Veterinary Surgery* 42: 544–550.

25 Steelman-Szymeczek, S.M., Stebbins, M.E., and Hardie, E.M. (2003). Clinical evaluation of a right-sided prophylactic gastropexy via a grid approach. *Journal of the American Animal Hospital Association* 39: 397–402.

26 Staiger, B.A., Stanley, B.J., and McAnulty, J.F. (2011). Single paracostal approach to the thoracic duct and cisterna chyle: experimental study and case series. *Veterinary Surgery* 40: 786–794.

27 Beittenmiller, M.R., Mann, F.A., Constantinescu, G.M. et al. (2009). Clinical anatomy and surgical repair of prepubic hernia in dogs and cats. *Journal of the American Animal Hospital Association* 45 (6): 284–290.

28 Tobias, K. (2017). *Manual of Small Animal Soft Tissue Surgery*, 2e. John Wiley & Sons, Inc.

Index